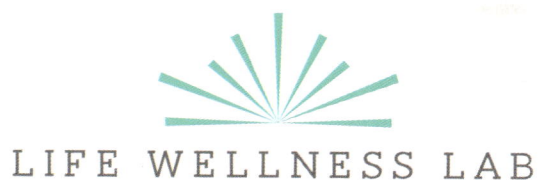

LIFE WELLNESS LAB

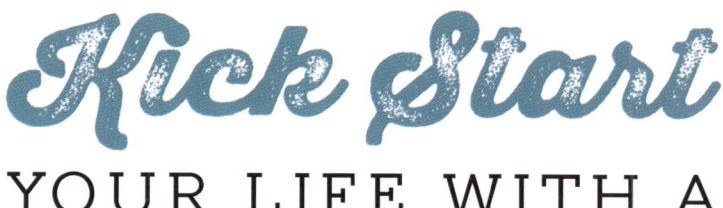

Kick Start

YOUR LIFE WITH A

14-DAY DETOX
CLEANSE

MELISSA MCLANE

WWW.LIFEWELLNESSLAB.COM

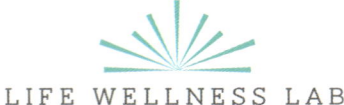

LIFE WELLNESS LAB

Published in July, 2018
by Life Wellness Lab
San Diego, CA
email: melissa@lifewellnesslab.com
www.lifewellnesslab.com

TABLE OF CONTENTS

Introduction

Welcome to this kickstart program to get you on the path to a lifelong health-foundation plan. There is no need to white knuckle through this program and don't worry about being hungry. The intent is for you to form healthy habits. Habits are formed when an action becomes part of your regular activities and you do not need to think much about it.

I created this 14-day program because just about anyone can commit to this short time-frame. It's also enough time to reset your body and it is an opportunity to reduce inflammation, get your blood sugar balanced, lose some weight and create new habits that pave the way to discover the ideal way of eating to achieve your optimal health.

This cleanse is an invitation to become more mindful and build awareness about what is keeping your from ultimate health and wellness as well as to tap into consistent self-care practices.

As you progress through this workbook, get curious and step into the experience. Notice what feels good to you and what doesn't.

The goal is help you to understand that you have choices in your life and to realize just

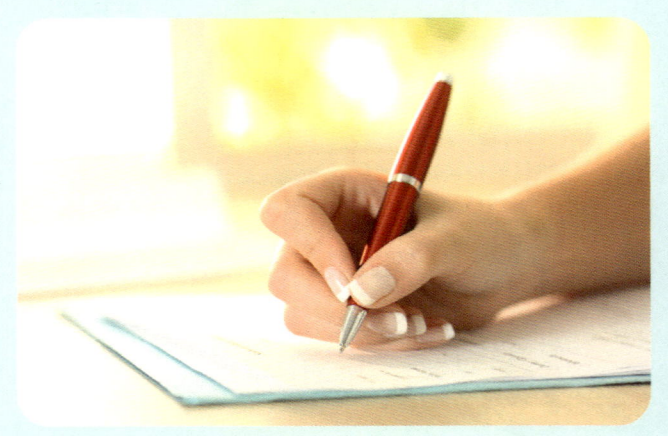

TIP: Journal daily
Studies have proven that journaling and writing down in your food journals have a 50% greater chance of succeeding. Prepare for success and be kind to yourself.

how important diet and lifestyle are in the management of prevention of disease, your vitality and longevity.

Don't feel as you have to make all the changes at once; it will take time and do just one thing at a time. Focus and give yourself permission to succeed. Start small, the smaller the better.

When making a plan look at the deeper reasons WHY; why do you want to make these changes, what are your excuses, what are your triggers, who is going to support you and what are your ways to be successful?

Pick your start date so you can prepare and you are giving yourself time to mentally and physically get ready. Build up anticipation and excitement. Plan a support system. Who will your turn to when you have a sugar craving, or when you have a strong urge? Do not underestimate the power of support – it is extremely important.

Benefits
- Shed excess weight
- Boost your energy
- Feel lighter and cleaner
- Decrease your craving for sugar
- Clearer skin
- Improve your gut health
- Create healthy habits
- Better mood
- Clearer, focused & improved mental state

I will walk you through some dietary changes as well as lifestyle changes that will combined promote healing, help you to start losing weight, reduce inflammation and balance your blood sugar.

Each system of the body relies on the others to keep the body functioning. Disease in one part of the body can disrupt and cause health problems in other parts of the body.

There is a direct link to gut health and healthy skin; weight gain and obesity to blood sugar imbalances; lifestyle to stress. Our bodies operate on many levels, therefore not one pill or one drug will solve your all of your symptom or health issues. There is no one bandaid approach. We need to take back our own health!

As a kid I was always curious and didn't understand how my grandmother could take 20+ pills a day and her doctors knew how all those pills affected her and her own unique biology. In my practice, I have seen miracles happen with my clients; by reversing diabetes, to clients that were plagued with migraines daily no longer have them, to clients that wanted to get back to their high school weight plus gain the same energy and playfulness as they did when they were a teenager.

This approach has my clients get off their medications and they are successful managing health issues and disease with diet and lifestyle. We can defy aging and live a younger youthful life even while we age. Living a long healthy life is ours.

Everyone's life is different and so is your biochemistry. Essentially you are not just what you eat, but you are also what you think. So your mindset plays a huge role in how you will succeed.

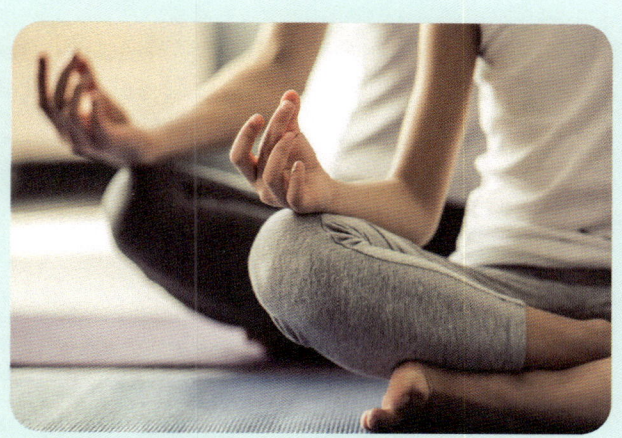

TIP: Self care
Take care of yourself – rest, stay hydrated, say no to things that are not good for you or take too much of your time. Stay away from people that bring you down or don't lift you up. Do not let any failure or guilt stop you from having what you want. They are just obstacles and you can overcome them. Regroup, let go, be kind to yourself, learn and get back up on that horse.

There is not one fool-proof diet/program that everyone should participate in to get the results they are looking for; however there are universal dietary principle everyone needs to follow if they want to lose fat, feel and be healthy and reverse or prevent chronic illnesses.

How to put all the pieces of the puzzle together? I like to think of this program a comprehensive set of recommendations that address the root cause of your symptoms.

Diet cannot work alone, stress management, adequate sleep, self care practices, and incorporating moderate physical activity into your life will improve the quality of your life.

Mindset

Be aware of how you talk to yourself. Start listening. When you start to notice and become aware of your inner voice, that is when you can start to make change permanently as those thoughts can derail any habit change.

It is important to discuss mindset and how we make excuses in our life for not having what we want. There is a section in this book that will allow you to dig into some of your excuses. How we do one thing is usually how we do everything in our life. So being able to look at your "WHYs" will hopefully shed some light into why you aren't healthy, fit, or where you want to be in your life.

On page 13, you will have an opportunity to really dig in and look at WHY. WHY do you want to be healthy now? WHY are you ready to make changes? What are your excuses?

Mindset roadblocks and where you get triggered are the most important to recognize. Try to identify if you have emotional eating patterns, you eat when you are bored, or eat when you feel stressed — these could be at a subconscious level and sabotage your success.

There are things you can do to change your mindset and prepare yourself for success. If you feel you do not think you can do this on your own, don't have enough support, or it is easier to eat the candy at work, or what if I am not perfect and I fail, or this is going to be hard — all these are just thoughts and

TIP: Fill out your trigger form so you can be aware of what gets you to fall off the rails.

TIP: Take some time to fill out the "Intake WHY form" – write down some of the things you tell yourself:

- I have to be perfect
- My life is harder than anyone else's
- I am too old
- It's not the right time
- I am too busy
- I am good enough
- I don't have enough support
- I don't know if I will succeed
- I don't have enough discipline
- I don't know if I can do it
- I go out to eat often and like to party

thoughts can be changed. You are in control of your own actions and thoughts. I promise you, you are fully capable of doing this program.

If you fall off track then tell yourself, "this food is not special, I can have it later if I decide I want it". You can have anything you want, just chose what is best for you and your goals in the moment. If you truly want to lose weight, then make that your priority and follow through with your actions.

As Tony Robbins says: "Change happens when the pain of staying the same is greater than the pain of change. At any moment, the decisions you make can change the course of your life forever."

Tips for a successful cleanse

There are several components to completing a successful detox cleanse. To make the next14-days a success, let's focus on ways to make small changes to your diet.

■ Introduce healthy fats: do not be afraid of eating healthy fats. by adding healthy fats you will feel full longer, you will reduce cravings, and promote healthy weight loss.

■ Increase your dark leafy greens; above ground vegetables including cruciferous vegetables.

■ Add fermented foods: it will help your gut health and reduce your cravings.

■ Drink enough water.

■ Get enough sleep: get 7-8 hours per night.

■ Gratitude: list 3 things each day before going to bed that you are so thankful for and practice taking a pause during the day to reflect on all the goodness in your life.

■ Exercise and move – daily.

■ Intermittent fast 1 or 2 days a week: last meal of the day 7 pm and first meal of the day 9 am.

■ De-clutter your pantry. Remove anything that will tempt you and get rid of all processed and junk food. Throw it all out, or donate to a home-less shelter.

■ Look at your labels and throw out: hydrogenated or partially hydrogenated oils.

TIP: Please note if you do not reduce your carbohydrate/sugar intake and increase you fat intake you will gain weight. Balancing your plate at each meal is important.

■ Buy organic, antibiotic- and hormone-free products: Free-range, meat and eggs, wild-caught fish.

■ Use high heat oils, coconut, MCT, avocado oil.

■ Use olive oil for low temperature cooking.

■ Throw out margarine. When buying nut butter, make sure the only ingredients are nuts, and salt (do not eat peanuts – they are legumes).

■ Avoid all soy products.

■ Say no to breads, pastas, sugars, pro-cessed foods, and other grains (these foods cause inflammation).

■ Options for sweeteners: coconut sugar or Stevia™ (do not eat artificial sweeteners, agave, Truvia™, Splenda™, white or brown sugar).

■ Add spices to your meals. Spices can help boost your metabolism.

■ Turn off all electronics, TV, cell phones, and computers at least an hour before bed. This will help to transition you into a good nights sleep.

■ Journal each day. Write down what foods you are eating so you can look back at what worked and where you can improve. Make small tweaks each day. Be diligent in writing everything you eat, what your mood is, how you feel. This is the only way to be able to really dig in and see the results you want. It takes each day to tweak your day, so you have lasting and greater results that last a lifetime.

Let's get started

4 Prep days

Here are the steps:

Prep Day 1: Read what foods you will be eating while on this program, what your plate should look like at each meal and look at what you need to avoid and that are off limits

Prep Day 2: Fill out your WHY and Trigger form, be committed to YOU and to your goals, why are you taking care of your health now? Commit and let the world know.

Prep Day 3: Clear your pantry and go shopping. Prep your foods and pick a day each week to plan what you will be eating and doing in that week, prep, go shopping.

Prep Day 4: Print out Fill out your measurements and weight form. Weigh yourself every week and continue even after the 14 days. Track your progress!

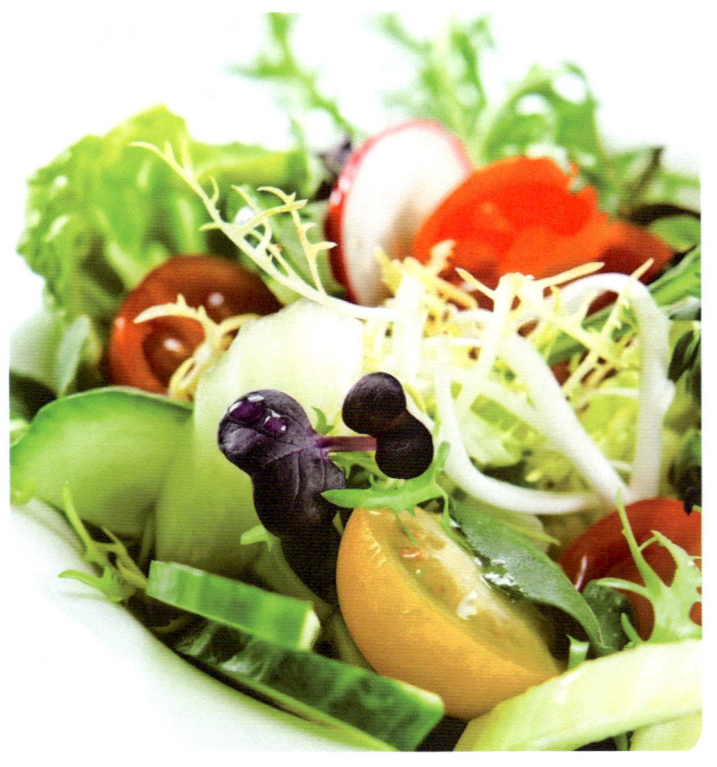

TIP: Setting your goals and determine your WHY is important. Once you start to see your success, your confidence will rise. You are not alone, feeling scared about doing a cleanse or feeling you are not capable are all normal feelings. The positive effects will be that you will start to lose weight, have more energy, think clearer and so much more. The best part is that you will start to gain more confidence as you see your results.

TIP: You can eat an abundant variety of delicious, satisfying foods to nurture both your physical and mental health. You will not go hungry or feel deprived. You can do this and it is worth it.

If you have a lot of plans and celebrations then plan on how you will make your decisions, what you will order and what you will eat based on the "allowed" foods.

Your actions and decisions will be the main factor of your success; how will you follow through, how will you prepare for traveling, or social gatherings. And so on.

What to eat/not to eat

Don't EAT:
- All grains, including gluten products
- Dairy
- Processed sugar
- Soy
- Soda, alcohol
- Safflower and corn oil
- Legumes and beans
- Corn peanuts

Optimal protein sources:
- Chicken and turkey
- Lamb, beef and wild game
- Eggs
- Shrimp
- Salmon, cod, trout and halibut
- Clams, mussels and oyster

Oils and fats
- Avocados
- Grass-fed butter and ghee
- Olive oil and olives
- Coconut
- Tahini
- Sesame seed oil
- Flax seed oil
- Raw nuts seeds and nut butters. (use sparingly)

Optimal super foods
- Hemp milk
- Goji berries
- Maca root
- Spirulina
- Chlorella

Gut healing foods:
- Aloe vera
- Bone broth
- Coconut
- Coconut yogurt
- Kimchi
- Kefir (raw and no sugar)
- Sauerkraut

Optimal fruit choices
- Avocados
- Berries
- Coconut meat oil and butter
- Granny Smith apples
- Lemons and limes

Optimal beverage choices
- Green veggies juice (no fruit added)
- Tea – organic
- Water – you can add lemon to flavor

Optimal carbohydrates:
- Arugula
- Asparagus
- Avocado
- Sprouts – Bean, alfalfa, broccoli,
- Beet greens
- Bok choy
- Broad beans
- Broccoli
- Brussels sprouts
- Cabbage, red and green
- Cauliflower
- Celery
- Chicory
- Chives
- Collard greens
- Dandelion greens
- Endive
- Escarole
- Fennel
- Garlic
- Ginger root
- Cilantro
- Kale
- Lettuces
- Mushrooms
- Onions
- Parsley
- Radish
- Seaweed
- Shallots
- Snow peas
- Spinach
- Swiss chard

Add a little spice to your life!
The 7 best spices

Cinnamon— can have many extreme benefits for improving heart disease and cutting the risk for diabetes, cancer as well as positive effects on blood sugar. Cinnamon adds sweetness without extra calories to drinks and desserts. A little bit of cinnamon goes a long way, and its antioxidant abilities are what makes it especially beneficial to include in your diet.

Cayenne pepper — has many medicinal benefits; it can be used to help digestion, stop stomach pain and is a natural remedy for cramps. It can improve poor circulation and lower high cholesterol. It can be used for a rub for meat and poultry and adds some heat to sauces and marinades.

Ginger — has been known for a wonderful alternative medicine to help digestion, reduce nausea and help fight the flu and common cold. It is good to add a spicy kick to baking and desserts, savory sauces and as a spice rub for meat.

Nutmeg — is a popular spice that has many health benefits; which include relieving pain, detoxifying the body, increasing skin health, reducing insomnia and improveing blood circulation. Nutmeg is often found in dessert sauces and baked goods, it also rounds out the flavor in savory sauces or can be sprinkled on grilled veggies

Garlic — by adding garlic to your diet, it has been known to boost the immune system and reduce the amount of sick days. Use fresh cloves to add zest to sauces, use garlic powder as a dry rub for meat, mix into burger patties or sprinkle on popcorn in lieu of salt.

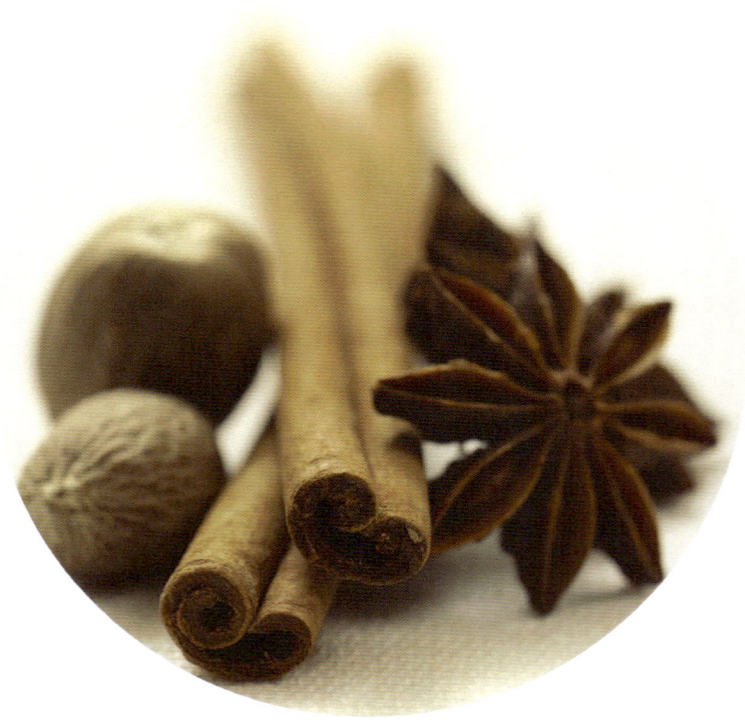

Cumin — the health benefits of cumin include its ability to aid in digestion, insomnia, respiratory disorders, asthma, bronchitis, common cold, lactation, anemia, and skin disorders. Adding cumin gives a smoky, spicy kick to soups, chili or stir-frys. Add it to ground turkey for spicy turkey tacos.

Saffron — is used to help loosen phlegm and for insomnia. Women can use it for menstrual cramps and PMS symptoms. Saffron lends a sweet and pungent zip to curry sauces and rice dishes, or add some to Greek yogurt for a sweet treat.

Helpful Supplements

Vitamin D

Vitamin D is needed to absorb calcium from the intestines; that's why it is so important for healthy bones. But vitamin D also appears to reduce the risk of various neuromuscular problems, particularly falling, and some preliminary evidence holds out hope that good levels of vitamin D may help reduce the risk of prostate cancer and certain other malignancies and perhaps of autoimmune diseases.

Resveratrol

May have numerous benefits such as lowering blood sugar levels and since it is considered an antioxidant and researchers found it can lower their LDL and increase HDL. Several studies have suggested it can protect the brain and decreases inflammation and suppress cancer cells. Resveratrol is a powerful antioxidant with great potential.

L-Theanine (Amino Acid)

L-Theanine is known to calm down the nervous systems to reduce stress. It produces a calming effect on the body. This amino acid is found primarily in black tea and green tea. Some people use L-Theanine for treating anxiety and high blood pressure. Scientists have known for years that when we are stressed we elevate cortisol levels, which interfere with learning, memory, lower immune function and bone density, increased weight gain, blood pressure, heart disease and the list goes on. The goal is to interrupt the fight or flight responds to everyday stressors, which creates adrenal imbalance and sometimes adrenal burnout.

DHEA-25

Dhea-25 is a hormone that is naturally produced by the adrenal glands. DHEA can help improve bone density, protects against depression, cognitive decline and mood swings. It aids in weight loss and building muscle mass and improves heart health, lower diabetes risk and decreases sexual dysfunction and can improve libido.

Coenzyme Q-10 (CoQ-10)

Supports heart health, reducing high blood pressure and cholesterol.

Glutamine (Amino Acid)

Supports digestive health and may help strengthen the immune system.

Probiotics

Probiotics can boost the immune system and promote intestinal health. When our gut is unhealthy we can expect other issues in our body to arise. What is needed is to remove problem foods and toxins and start to heal and repair the gut by eating a clean diet. With the addition of probiotics, we can begin to restore the ideal balance of bacteria and maintain new optimal health.

Omega-3 fats

Help lower cholesterol and may positively impact learning and brain health as well as reduce the risk of heart disease.

Curcumin

Curcumin Is a very powerful anti-aging, anti-inflammatory and anti-cancer spice. It's a powerful antioxidant and improves brain function. It can help depression and eases arthritis. It can be used to treat cancer, slows the process of aging and helps manage insulin levels.

MCT Oil

Helps to maintain a healthy weight. Specifically reduces stored body fat, because it raises your metabolic function. Helps you have more energy and think more clearly, experience better digestion, balances hormone levels and improves your mood.

Collagen and Peptides

Support balanced hormones, bone and joint health, digestion and satiety. Good for the skin, hair and nails. They also help with joint pain, promote better sleep, keep bones strong, improve digestion, help lose weight and reduce inflammation.

Bone Broth

It's packed with collagen and is found to be a pretty potent natural skin care product. Also, helps to keep our joints moving without pain. Bone broth is great for your gut as it's a probiotic and keeps inflammation in the digestive track at bay and supports intestinal health.

Getting to know your symptoms

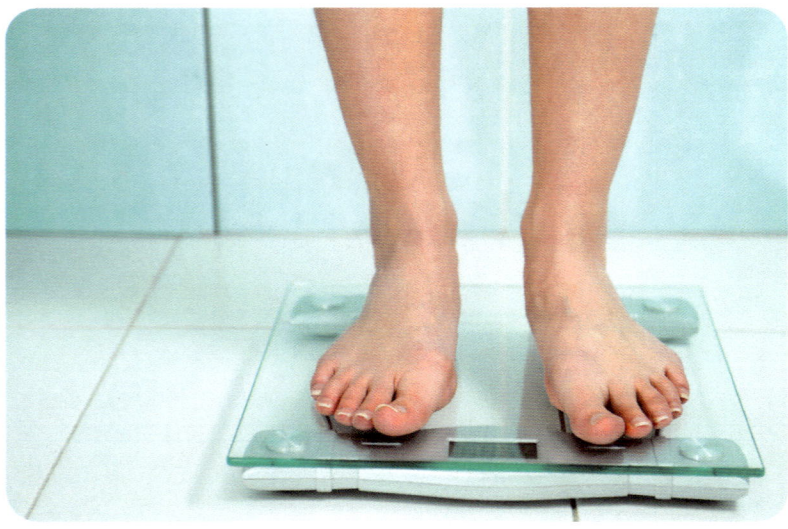

If you answered YES to most of these questions then balancing your blood sugar is our first line of defense. If you primary goal is to lose weight, but you have a lot of other lifestyle stressors it is important to follow this book to the best of your ability.

This program doesn't just eliminate sweeteners and sugary processed foods, it also eliminates some of the most common food allergens; gluten, soy, corn, and (for some) dairy.

This program gives your body a break and relief from some of the potential irritants.

Current weight

Ideal goal weight

Are there foods you avoid because how they make you feel? **Yes / No**

Do you have immediate symptoms? (gas bloating?) **Yes / No**

Do you crave sweets or carbs in the afternoon or evening? **Yes / No**

Must have sweets after a meal? **Yes / No**

Difficulty losing weight? **Yes / No**

I do not get a good nights sleep **Yes / No**

Cannot fall asleep **Yes / No**

Headaches **Yes / No**

Wake up tired even after 6 hours of sleep **Yes / No**

TIP: Enlist support. Invest in a coach and if you can't enlist your friends to support you through your change. It is always easier when people around you are going through this with you. A health coach can cheer you on, make adjustments to what you're doing — just like for an athlete or someone wanting to start a business. Having your own personal coach who is there to fully support you is a path for success. Your coach will keep you accountable and is important for your success. While many people complete this program without any additional help, if you find yourself needing a little extra support, contact melissa@lifewellnesslab.com.

Your Why

Use the space below to write down your WHY.

1. Why is improving your health important to you?

_____

_____

_____

2. Why now?

_____

_____

_____

3. What are some common thoughts you have about:

your body?

_____

your job?

_____

your significant relationship?

_____

your financial state?

_____

5. Nutrition: Will you follow this guide for the next 14 days?

_____

_____

_____

4. Goals:

Daily movement/exercise goal:

_____

Weekly movement/exercise goal:

_____

How many hours of sleep/night:

_____

What will you do when you feel stressed? (_breathe, walk, get support from a friend_)

_____

_____

_____

_____

Commitment signature to your goals:

X_____

Baseline Body Measurements

Body Measurements can be a useful way to track your progress. Many times you will see lost in inches even if the scale is not moving. To ensure accuracy, measure in exactly the same place and under the same conditions each time.

WEEK 1   **WEEK 6**

Calculate your body mass index (BMI):
Go to: https://www.nhlbi.nih.gov/health/educational/lose_wt/BMI/bmicalc.htm

BUST: Place the measuring tape across your nipples and measure around the largest part of your chest. (Be sure to keep the tape parallel)

WEEK 1	WEEK 2	WEEK 3	WEEK 4	WEEK 5	WEEK 6

CHEST: Place the measuring tape just under your breasts/pectorals and measure around the torso while keeping the tape parallel to the floor.

WEEK 1	WEEK 2	WEEK 3	WEEK 4	WEEK 5	WEEK 6

WAIST: Place the measuring tape about a 1/2 inch above your bellybutton (at the narrowest part of your waist) to measure around your torso. When measuring your waist, exhale and measure before inhaling again.

WEEK 1	WEEK 2	WEEK 3	WEEK 4	WEEK 5	WEEK 6

HIPS: Place the measuring tape across the widest part of your hips/buttocks and measure all the way around while keeping the tape parallel to the floor.

WEEK 1	WEEK 2	WEEK 3	WEEK 4	WEEK 5	WEEK 6

WEIGHT:

WEEK 1	WEEK 2	WEEK 3	WEEK 4	WEEK 5	WEEK 6

NOTES:_____

Honoring Hunger & Fullness

If you want to build healthy habits around food, what you eat is only part of the big picture. We also have to look at:

- HOW we eat
- Do you eat when you're not actually hungry?
- Do you eat too little or too much?

How do we "Honor Hunger"?

- Tune into your internal signal that the body needs nourishment
- Recognize hunger - learn the signs
- Create an intuitive inner scale from 1-10
- 1 is just noticing hunger, 10 is starving
- Start to plan for food when you are at a 2

How do we "Honor Fullness"?

- Create a fullness scale from 1-10
- 10 is stuffed, 1 is still starving
- Aim for a 7 on the fullness scale - nourished and energized, satiated but not stuffed

(Hunger scale thermometer diagram: 10 = STARVING, PLAN FOR FOOD at 2, NOTICING HUNGER at 1, labeled HUNGER SCALE)

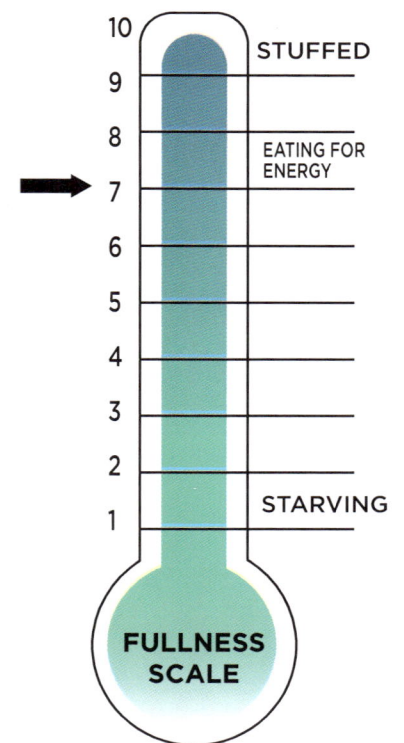

Logically, the hunger and fullness scale make sense. Start planning when you are at level 2 on the hunger scale and stop eating when you are at level 7 on the fullness scale. Here's the problem, most of us have habits of eating beyond fullness. So let's create some new habits around honoring hunger and fullness.

1. Start planning what and when to eat when you are at a level 2.

2. Eat high-energy foods that your body wants.

3. Eat for energy (level 7 on the fullness scale).

4. Make a physical gesture that your meal is complete by pushing your plate away, putting a napkin over it, or crossing silverware.

5. Declare out loud to yourself or whomever you are eating with that you are full. This will dissuade you from continuing to eat because you've already announced that the meal was complete for you.

6. If you're out, ask your server to box up the rest of the meal so it's not calling you hither.

Honoring Hunger and Fullness: Courtesy of Health Coach Institute

Trigger Form

Physical Triggers: How have these common physical triggers for overeating affected you? What strategies can you come up with to deal with each trigger more effectively?

❒ Thirst

❒ Fatigue

❒ Urge to chew, crunch or suck

❒ Pain

❒ Hormonal cycles

❒ Medical conditions

_____

_____

_____

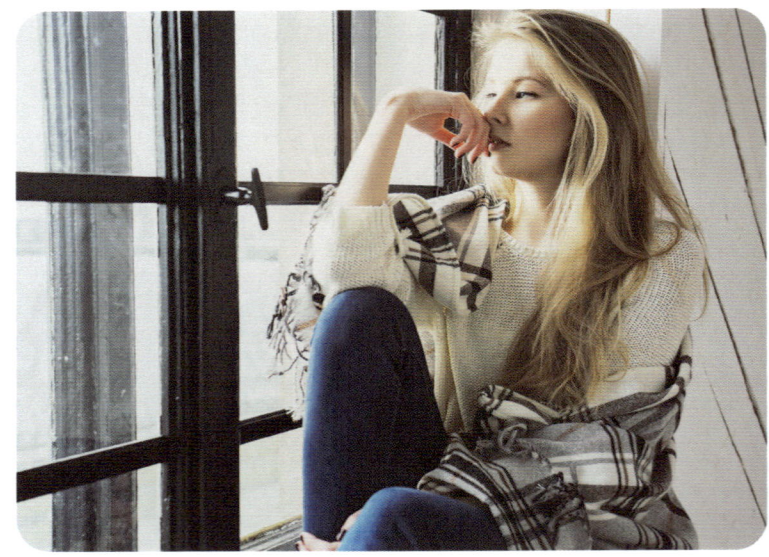

Environmental: Common cues for overeating include people, places, activities, and events that you associate with eating. Be creative when coming up with strategies for dealing with these common triggers.

❒ Mealtimes

❒ Eating on a schedule

❒ High-risk times

❒ Holidays

❒ Weather

❒ Preventing eating

❒ Grocery shopping

❒ Advertising

❒ Social events

❒ Watching TV

❒ Dining out

❒ Eating at work

❒ Entertaining

❒ Mindless eating

Emotional: Identify emotions that trigger a desire to eat (including specific examples). Brainstorm better ways to distract, calm, comfort, and nurture yourself without turning to food.

❒ Pleasure

❒ Reward

❒ Love

❒ Boredom

❒ Stress

❒ Feeling Overwhelmed

❒ Loneliness

❒ Worry and Tension

❒ Sadness

❒ Avoidance

❒ Guilt and Shame

❒ Anger

❒ Negative Self Talk

❒ Perfectionist thinking

❒ Restriction and Deprivation

❒ Diets

❒ Negative body image

❒ Weighing yourself

❒ Eating Disorder

Hydration

Getting enough water every day is important for your health. Water acts as a catalyst for renewal, like when you water plants and watch them grow. Drink at least 64 ounces (8- 8 oz glasses) of water daily. Water helps regulate your body temperature, aids in digestion, metabolism, prevents constipation, helps to maintain healthy muscles and supports your organs.

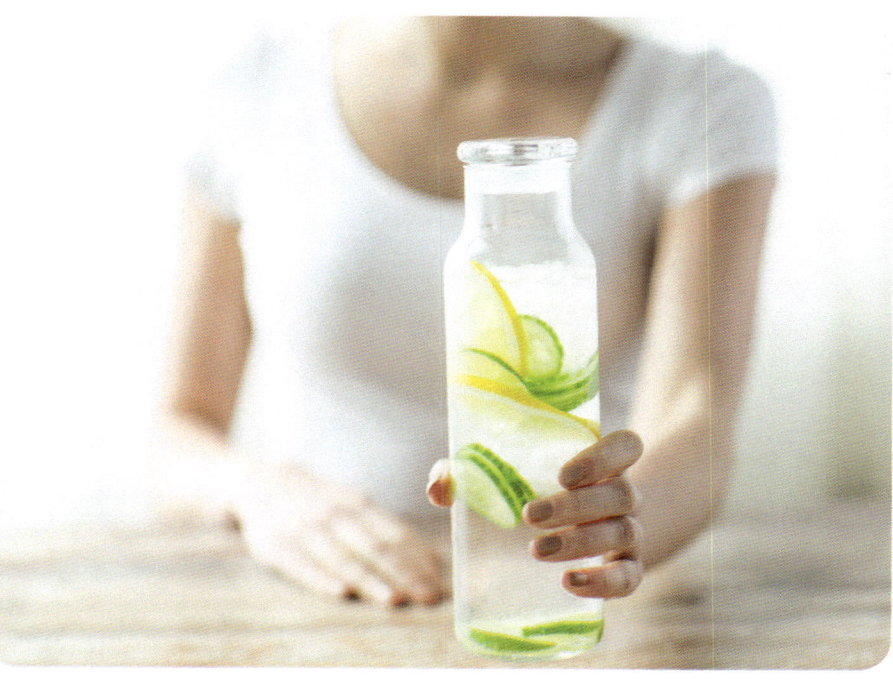

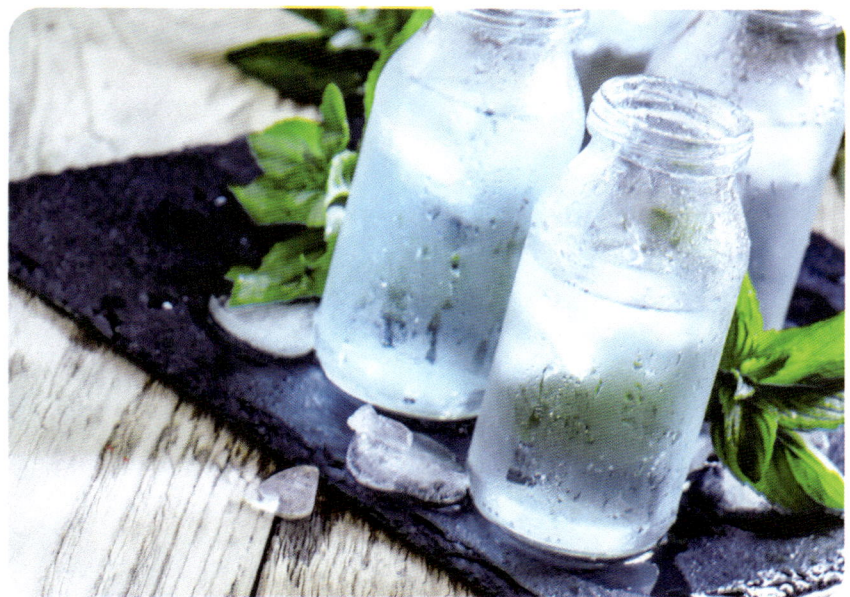

Moderate Dehydration Symptoms:

- Dry, sticky mouth
- Dizziness or lightheadedness
- Dry skin
- Headache

Severe Dehydration Symptoms

- A rapid weak pulse
- Rapid breathing
- Confusion
- Lack of sweating

TIP

The success on this cleanse will be in direct correlation with how much you believe in yourself and that you can make decisions and take control of your life and health.

Disclaimer: The author is not a physician and does not offer any medical diagnoses or treatments

Plate Distribution

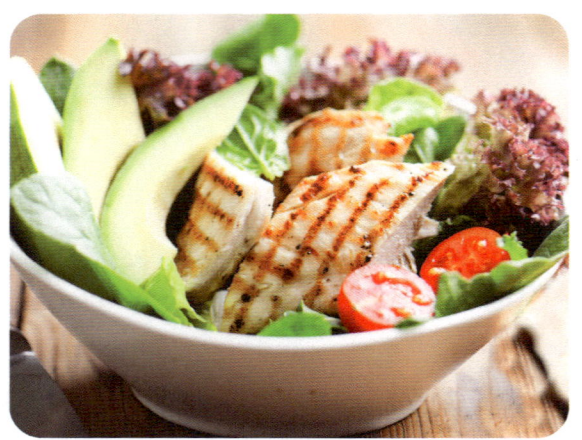

20-30%
NON-starchy veggies
Have at least 2 or more
servings at every meal
(1/2 cup cooked + 1 cup raw)

35%-40%
Healthy Fats
(FAT does not make you fat)
2-3 servings of healthy fat
at every meal.

35%-40%
Lean Protein
Every meal includes
1 serving of protein 4-6 oz.

8 Snack Ideas

1. Two hard boiled eggs with salt

2. Two tablespoons almond butter on celery stick (try Wholefoods 365 brand)

3. Two turkey roll-ups: slice of avocado, slice of cucumber, roll sliced turkey around it

4. Two roast beef roll ups: goat cheese, slice of red pepper, roll roast beef slice around

5. 4 oz wild salmon or beef jerky

6. Protein shake: almond milk, cinnamon, spinach, protein powder (optional: cacao powder, chia seeds)

7. Half a cup of guacamole and crudités (cucumber, carrots, peas, etc.)

8. Half an avocado with a little olive oil and salt

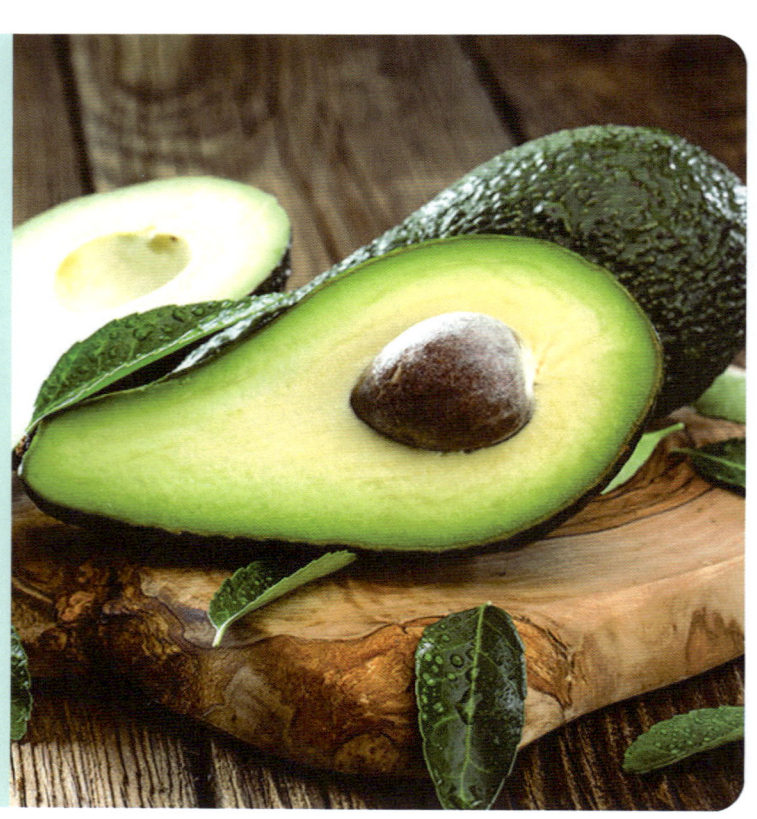

Week 1

Breakfast:

- **Monday:** Caramelized chicken hash with brussels sprouts

- **Tuesday:** Scrambled eggs with bacon and vegetables

- **Wednesday:** Smoothie

- **Thursday:** Chicken breakfast sausage

- **Friday:** Simple frittata

- **Saturday:** Eggs & vegetables, fried in coconut oil

- **Sunday:** Smoothie

Lunch/Snack:

- **Monday:** Cabbage with bacon

- **Tuesday:** Detox salad

- **Wednesday:** Chicken chili

- **Thursday:** Leftover chicken chili

- **Friday:** Leftover spaghetti squash "pasta"

- **Saturday:** Left over asian cabbage stir-fry

- **Sunday:** Go-to chicken salad roll-ups

Dinner

- **Monday:** Chicken chili

- **Tuesday:** Spaghetti squash "pasta"

- **Wednesday:** Asian cabbage stir-fry

- **Thursday:** Citrus fish tacos

- **Friday:** Zucchini and fennel soup

- **Saturday:** Bacon burgers

- **Sunday:** Pork meatloaf

Shopping list

Grilled chicken	Spaghetti squash
Shallots	Carrots
Zucchini	Celery
Garlic	Mushrooms
Spinach	Red wine vinegar
Turkey bacon	Ground thyme
Zucchini	Oregano
Parsley	Basil
Sage	Can of tuna
Garlic powder	Chives
Onion powder	Lettuce leaves
Black pepper	Mayo (avocado oil)
Dried thyme	Red onion
Red pepper flakes	Red grapes
Ground nutmeg	Almonds
MCT oil	Tahini

Grass-fed butter
Ground cloves
Eggs
Ground chicken or ground beef
Broccoli
Coconut milk
Cauliflower
Shredded cabbage
Bacon
Chicken
Tamari
Lemons
Almond milk *(or coconut milk* look on smoothie recipe options)*
Sesame oil
Miso
Pecans
Onion
Bell pepper
Chili powder
Cumin
Coriander
Diced tomatoes
Bone broth
Lime
Cilantro
Coconut oil or avocado oil

Week 2

Breakfast

- **Monday:** Veggies and egg muffins
- **Tuesday:** Smoothie
- **Wednesday:** Chicken breakfast sausage
- **Thursday:** Eggs & vegetables, fried in coconut oil
- **Friday:** Scrambled eggs with bacon and vegetables
- **Saturday:** Sausages with sliced avocado and spinach
- **Sunday:** smoothie

Lunch/Snack

- **Monday:** Leftover baked salmon with pesto, lemon & dill
- **Tuesday:** Leftover yummy vinegar dressing, chicken stir fry
- **Wednesday:** Smoothie
- **Thursday:** Leftover chicken chili
- **Friday:** Go-to chicken salad roll-ups
- **Saturday:** Smoothie
- **Sunday:** Citrus fish tacos

Dinner

- **Monday:** Baked salmon with pesto, lemon & dill
- **Tuesday:** Yummy vinegar dressing, chicken stir fry
- **Wednesday:** Chicken chili
- **Thursday:** Zucchini and fennel soup
- **Friday:** Pork meatloaf
- **Saturday:** Coconut lamb with cauliflower rice
- **Sunday:** Ground turkey tacos

Shopping list

Sausage
Coconut oil
Spinach
Mushrooms
Avocado
Green onion
Wild caught fish
*smoothie ingredients
Lamb
Onion
Carrot
Tomatoes
Zucchini
Coconut mild / cream
Cilantro
Cauliflower rice
Spinach
MCT, avocado oil, coconut oil
Seasonings (garlic, salt, pepper, ginger, etc)
Lemon
Lime
Mushrooms
Eggs
Chicken bone broth
Fennel bulb
Blueberries / strawberries
Lettuce leaves
Red onion
Mango
Red pepper
Almonds or walnuts
Chicken
Grapes
Sesame oil
cabbage
Wasabi paste
Fresh ginger
Chili flakes
Ground beef
Oranges

Breakfast Recipes

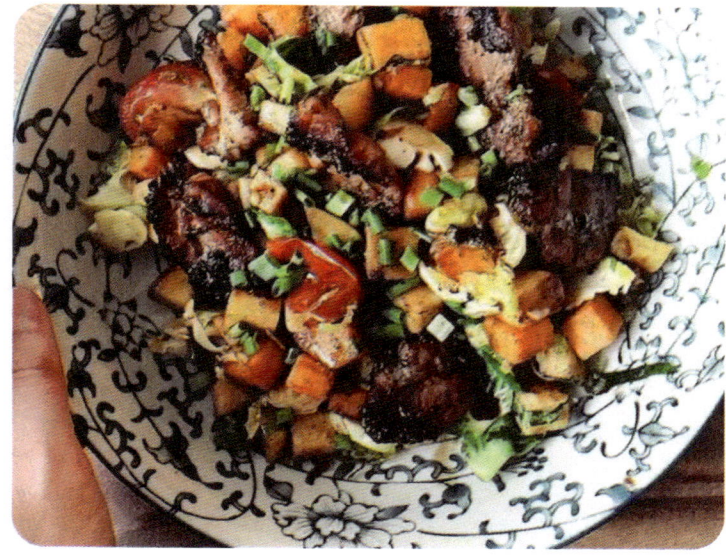

Caramelized Chicken Hash with Brussels Sprouts

Serves: 4
Cooking time: 20 minutes
Meal: Breakfast

Ingredients

1 cup grilled chicken
1 Tbsp shallots
1 medium zucchini, diced
1 clove garlic, minced
Large handful of spinach
Tablespoons of coconut oil, avocado oil, or MTC oil

Instructions

Slice the cooked grilled chicken into bite sizes. Heat 1 Tbsp coconut oil over medium-high heat in a sauté pan. When hot add chicken and shallots sauté until cooked through. Add zucchini and Brussels sprouts, garlic, and spinach and season with a small pinch of salt and black pepper. Keep stir-frying for an additional 2 minutes. Serve hot and enjoy!

Scrambled Eggs with Bacon and Vegetables

Serves: 2
Cooking time: 20 minutes
Meal: Breakfast

Ingredients

4 slices turkey bacon
4 eggs
1 medium zucchini, diced
1 clove garlic, minced
1 medium tomato, diced
Large handful of spinach
1 tbsp of coconut oil, avocado oil, or MTC oil

Instructions

Cook bacon - remove from pan. Chop vegetables. Over medium-high heat, add zucchini, garlic, and tomato to the pan with oil. Sauté until tender. Beat eggs in small bowl. Crumble bacon and set aside.
When vegetables are almost done, add the beated eggs and crumbled bacon to the pan, along with fresh spinach. Turn heat to med-low and cook until eggs are fluffy and firm.

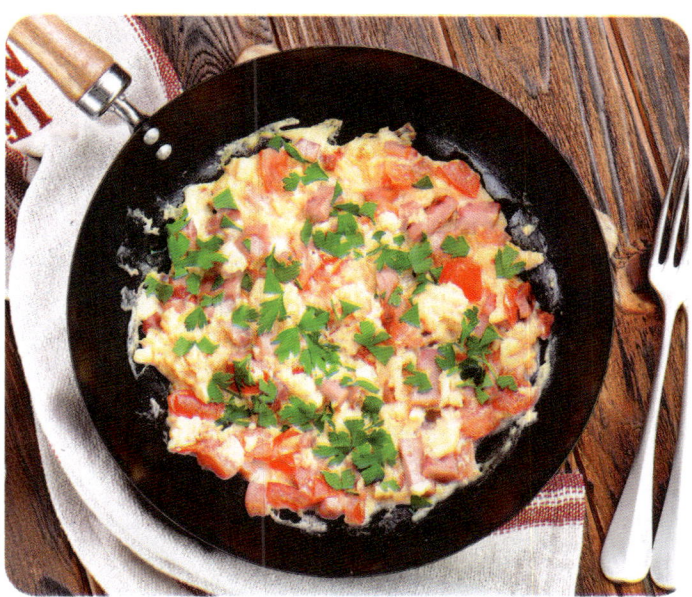

Chicken Breakfast Sausage

Serves: 8 (2 patties per serving)

Cooking time: 30 minutes

Meal: Breakfast

Ingredients

2 lbs. ground chicken or ground beef

2 tsp. Himalayan pink salt

2 tsp. rubbed sage

1 1/2 tsp. dried parsley

1 tsp. garlic powder

1 tsp. onion powder

1 tsp. black pepper

1/2 tsp. dried thyme

1/4 tsp. red pepper flakes

1/4 tsp. ground nutmeg

Healthy fat (*MCT, ghee, grass-fed butter, coconut oil*)

Pinch ground cloves

Instructions

In a large mixing bowl, combine ground chicken, salt, rubbed sage, parsley, garlic powder, onion powder, black pepper, thyme, red pepper flakes, nutmeg, and cloves. Mix until all ingredients are well mixed. Roll them into balls and then flatten them into patties. Heat a large skillet over medium heat. Oil the skillet. Once the oil is heated, place the sausage patties in the pan. Cook until browned on both sides and cooked all the way through.

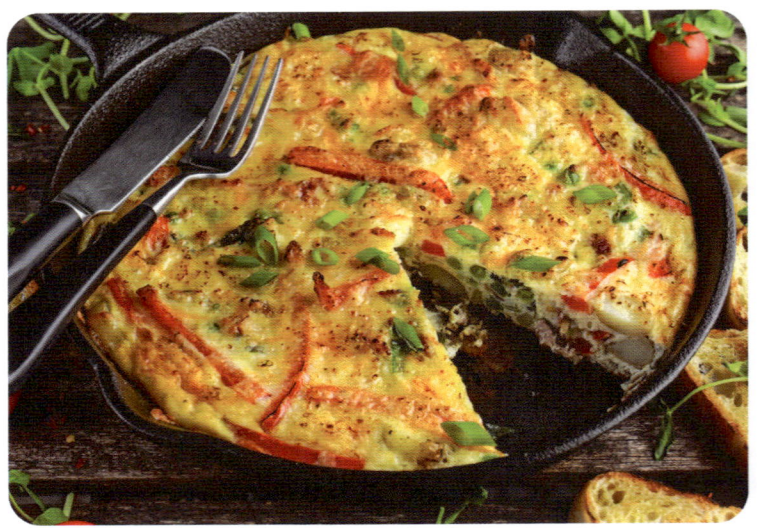

Simple Frittata

Serves: 2

Cooking time: 25 minutes

Meal: Breakfast

Ingredients

1 Tbsp coconut oil or healthy fat of choice

1 cup Protein (whatever cooked meat you have on hand)

1 cup broccoli

2 Tbsp coconut milk

4 eggs

Salt and pepper to taste

Instructions

Preheat the toaster oven to 350°F and heat the coconut oil in an 8-inch cast iron skillet over medium heat. Add protein to the skillet and stir-fry until heated through. Cut the broccoli into bite-sized pieces. Crack the eggs into a medium bowl, and add the coconut milk, salt, and a few grinds of pepper. Whisk well. Pour the egg mixture into the skillet and cook for 3 to 5 minutes or until the bottom of the frittata is set. Place the skillet in the oven. Cook for 10 to 15 minutes, and then crank the heat up to broil for another 2 minutes or until the frittata puffs up and is cooked all the way through.

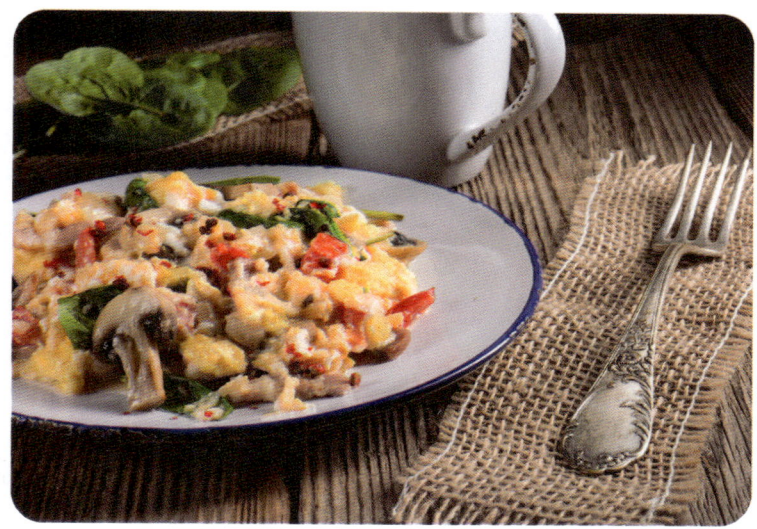

Eggs and Vegetables, Fried in Coconut Oil

Serves: 2

Cooking time: 15 minutes

Meal: Breakfast

Ingredients

2 Tbsp for coconut Oil

4 eggs

1 medium zucchini, diced

1 clove garlic, minced

1 cup cauliflower

2 cups of spinach

1 cup of broccoli

Assorted spices

Instructions

Add coconut oil into frying pan and turn up the heat Chop vegetables. Over medium-high heat, add veggies to the pan with oil. Sauté until tender. Beat eggs in small bowl. Turn heat to med-low and cook until eggs are fluffy and firm.

Sausages with Sliced Avocado and Spinach

Serves: 2

Cooking time: 15 minutes

Meal: Breakfast

Ingredients

1 sausage

1 Tbsp coconut or avocado oil

1 cup spinach

¼ cup onion

1 cup mushrooms

½ avocado sliced

Chopped green onion

Spices to taste

Instructions

Heat the oil in an 8-inch skillet over medium heat.

Add sausages, mushrooms, and onions to the skillet and stir-fry until heated through. Cook until done. Slice avocado and add on side.

Cabbage with Bacon

Serves: 2

Cooking time: 25 minutes

Meal: Breakfast

Ingredients

2 cups, shredded cabbage

4 slices bacon

salt and pepper to taste

Instructions

Fill a pot with just enough water to cover cabbage and boil cabbage for 5-7 minutes. Cook bacon and crumble. Add salt and bacon to cabbage and enjoy.

Lunch Recipes

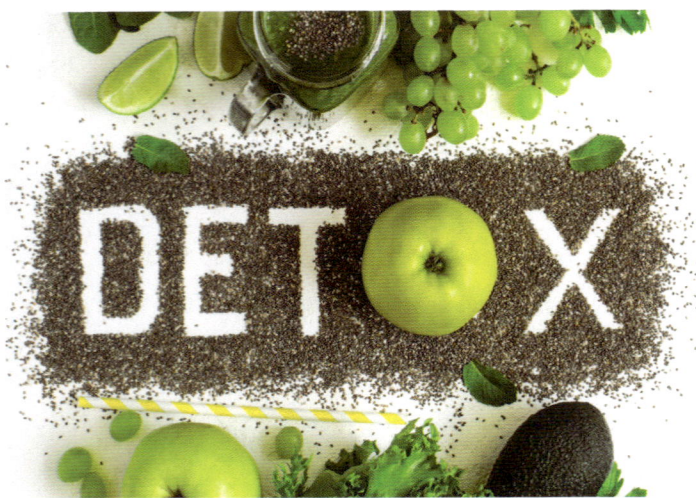

Detox Salad

Serves: 2

Cooking time: 15 minutes

Meal: Lunch

Ingredients

1 tablespoon coconut oil

1 cup shredded cabbage

1 1/2 cups broccoli florets, finely chopped

1 1/2 cups cauliflower florets, finely chopped

1 clove garlic, minced

8 oz chopped chicken

3 tbsp low sodium tamari

3 tbsp lemon juice

2 tsp sesame oil

1 tbsp miso (optional)

sea salt and pepper, to taste

1/4 cup chopped toasted pecans

Instructions

Heat the oil in a saute pan over medium heat. Add the cabbage, broccoli, cauliflower and garlic. Cook for 4-5 minutes to soften. In a small bowl, whisk together the tamari, lemon juice, sesame oil and miso. Pour over the cabbage mix and mix to combine. Season with salt and pepper. Take off the heat and mix in the chopped pecans.

Chicken Chili

Serves: 4

Cooking time: 25 minutes

Meal: Lunch

Ingredients

2 tablespoons avocado oil

1 yellow onion, diced

3 cloves garlic, peeled and minced

1 red bell pepper, diced

1 green bell pepper, diced

2 teaspoons chili powder

1 teaspoon ground cumin

1 teaspoon ground coriander

1/4 teaspoon red pepper flakes

1 teaspoon sea salt, more to taste

1 28 ounce jar diced tomatoes (no sugar added)

1 cup chicken bone broth

2 cooked chicken breasts, diced

1 lime, cut into wedges

4 tablespoons chopped cilantro

Instructions

Heat the oil in a pot over medium heat. Add the onion, garlic and peppers and cook for 3-4 minutes. Add the spices, tomatoes, stock and chicken and cook for 15-20 minutes to allow the flavors to meld. Top with 1 tablespoon chopped cilantro and a lime wedge.

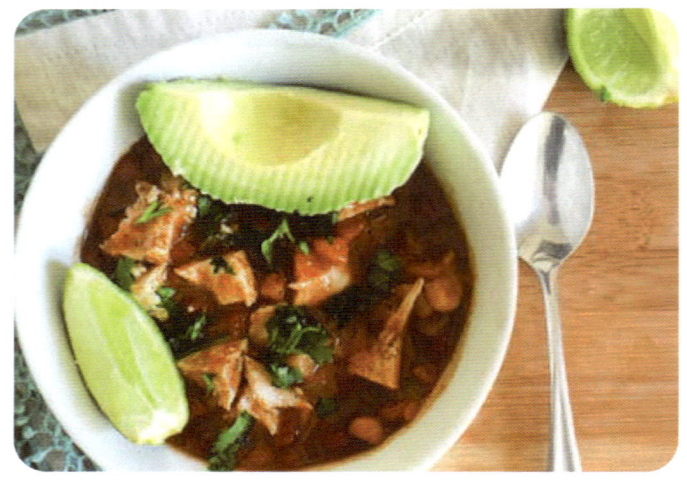

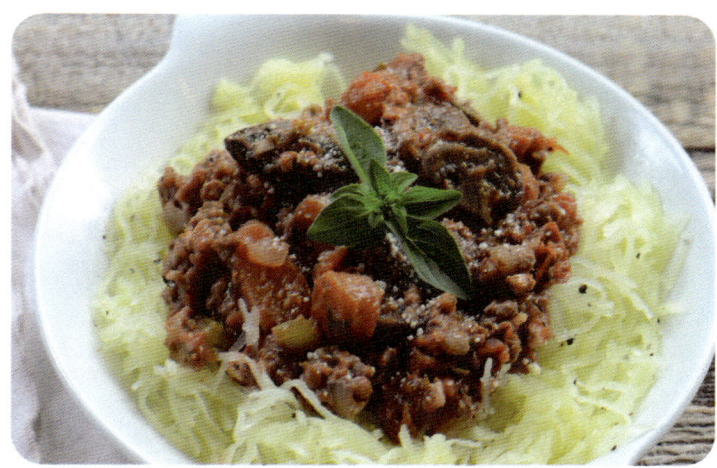

Spaghetti Squash Pasta

Serves: 4
Cooking time: 60 minutes
Meal: Lunch

Ingredients

2 spaghetti squash, cut in half and seeds removed
3 tbsp avocado, divided
1 yellow onion, diced
2 carrots, diced
3 celery stalks, diced
3 cloves garlic, peeled and minced
1 lb baby bella mushrooms, ends trimmed & diced
1 28 ounce jar crushed tomatoes
2 tablespoons red wine vinegar
1/2 teaspoon ground thyme
1 teaspoon dried oregano and basil
sea salt and pepper, to taste
Side Salad:
4 cups mixed greens dressing of choice

Instructions

Place 4 cups of water in a large pot. Add the spaghetti squash halves and bring the water to a boil. Cook the squash for 15-20 minutes or until fork tender. While the squash is cooking, start making the sauce. Heat 2 tablespoons of oil in a saute pan over medium heat. Add the onion, carrot, celery, garlic and mushrooms and cook for 3-4 minutes to soften. Add the crushed tomatoes, vinegar and spices. Cook for 10-15 minutes to allow the flavors to meld. When the spaghetti squash is done, take each half and scrape out the inside with a fork to create "spaghetti strands".

Go-To Chicken Salad Roll-Ups

Serves: 1
Cooking time: 15 minutes
Meal: Lunch

Ingredients

4-8 ounces chopped chicken breast (precooked)
2-3 Butter lettuce leaves
1/4 cup chopped almonds
5 red seedless grapes, halved
1/4 mashed avocado
Salt & pepper, to taste

Instructions

Mix all ingredients (minus the lettuce leaves) in a bowl. Spoon into butter lettuce leaves to make a nice wrap!

Canned Tuna mixed with Chives and Olive Oil Mayo

Serves: 2
Cooking time: 15 minutes
Meal: Lunch

Ingredients

1 can of tuna
A bunch of chives
Lettuce leaves
Avocado
Mayo (with avocado oil)
Red onion

Instructions

Open tuna can and drain liquids. Put in bowl and mix with Mayo, chopped chives, and red onion. Server inside of lettuce leaves and add avocado as garnish.

Asian Cabbage Stir-Fry

Serves: 4
Cooking time: 60 minutes
Meal: Lunch

Ingredients

1 2/3 lbs green cabbage
5 1/3 oz. butter
1 1/3 lbs ground beef
1 tsp salt
1 tsp onion powder
1/4 tsp ground black pepper
1 tbsp white wine vinegar
2 garlic cloves
3 scallions, in slices
1 tsp chili flakes
1 Tbsp fresh ginger, finely chopped or grated
1 Tbsp wasabi mayonnaise
1 cup mayonnaise
1/2 – 1 tablespoon wasabi paste

Instructions

Shred the cabbage nely using a sharp knife or a food processor. Fry the cabbage in 2–3 ounces (60–90 g) butter in a large frying or wok pan on medium-high heat, but don't let the cabbage turn brown. It takes a while for the cabbage to soften. Add spices and vinegar. Stir and fry for a couple of minutes more. Put the cabbage in a bowl. Melt the rest of the butter in the same frying pan. Add garlic, chili flakes and ginger and sauté for a few minutes. Add ground meat and brown until the meat is thoroughly cooked and most of the juices have evaporated. Lower the heat a little. Add scallions and cabbage to the meat. Stir until everything is hot. Add salt and pepper to taste, and top with the sesame oil before serving. Serve the stir-fry warm with a dollop of wasabi mayonnaise on top.

Bacon Burgers

Serves: 4
Cooking time: 60 min
Meal: Lunch

Ingredients

1/2 pound cremini mushrooms, thinly sliced
2 tbsp lard or fat of choice, divided
4 slices bacon, frozen
1 pound ground beef
1 1/2 tsp kosher salt
Freshly ground black pepper
4 leaves from a head of butter lettuce, rinsed & dried
1 large, ripe tomato, sliced

Instructions

Cut mushrooms into small pieces and cook in cast-iron skillet with half of the lard. Set aside mushrooms. Cut bacon into small strips (cutting frozen bacon is easiest). Mix mushrooms, bacon, and beef together with salt and pepper. Form 4 big patties (3/4 inch thick). Fry patty up in hot oil ~3 min per side. Wrap burgers in lettuce with tomato.

Zucchini and Fennel Soup

Serves: 3-4
Cooking time: 45 minutes
Meal: Lunch

Ingredients

1 tbsp. extra virgin olive oil
3 zucchini, chopped and peeled
1/2 onion, chopped
1/2 fennel bulb, chopped
3 cups chicken stock (low sodium)
Salt and pepper to taste

Instructions

Heat olive oil in a large skillet or soup pot with zucchini, onion, and chopped fennel.
Season with salt and pepper. Cook for about 10-15 min. Add stock, bring to a boil and then simmer until soft. Put everything in blender and blend. Serve immediately and enjoy!

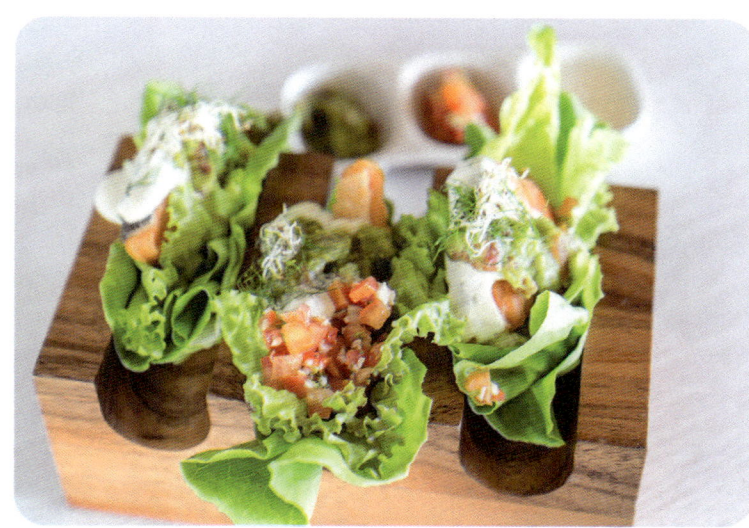

Citrus Fish Tacos

Serves: 2
Cooking time: 2-4 hours
Meal: Lunch

Ingredients

Marinade:
2 large oranges (juiced)
1/2 lime (juiced)
3 tbsp olive oil
1 tsp. cumin powder
1/2 tsp salt
2 wild-caught tilapia fillets (cut in 1" chunks)
Wraps:
3-6 butter lettuce leaves
1/2 red pepper (diced)
1/2 red onion (diced)
1/2 mango (diced)
1/2 avocado (sliced)

Instructions

Mix the orange juice, lime juice, olive oil, cumin, and salt in a bowl and combine well. Gently place the pieces of Tilapia into a large zipper bag and pour in the juice. Marinade for 2-4 hours in the refrigerator, flipping the bag over about half way through.

Egg Salad

Serves: 3-4
Cooking time: 45 minutes
Meal: Lunch

Ingredients

10 large eggs
4 ounces bacon, chilled in freezer for 20 minutes
1/3 cup homemade Paleo mayonnaise or Primal Kitchen Mayonnaise
1 tbsp Dijon mustard
2 tbsp fresh lemon juice
1 large shallot, minced (about ¼ cup)
¼ cup minced fresh Italian parsley leaves
2 tbsp minced fresh chives
1½ tsp Diamond Crystal brand kosher salt
¼ tsp ground black pepper
2 cups lettuce leaves (optional)
½ cup sprouts (optional)
Small sweet peppers (optional)

Instructions

Hard boil eggs. Slice bacon and render in a cast iron skillet (15-20 min). Peel eggs, cut into half lengthwise and pop out yolks into a bowl. Add mayo, mustard, lemon juice, into yolk bowl and stir and smush until mostly smooth. Roughly chop egg whites and add the rest of the ingredients. Stuff salad into sweet bell peppers!

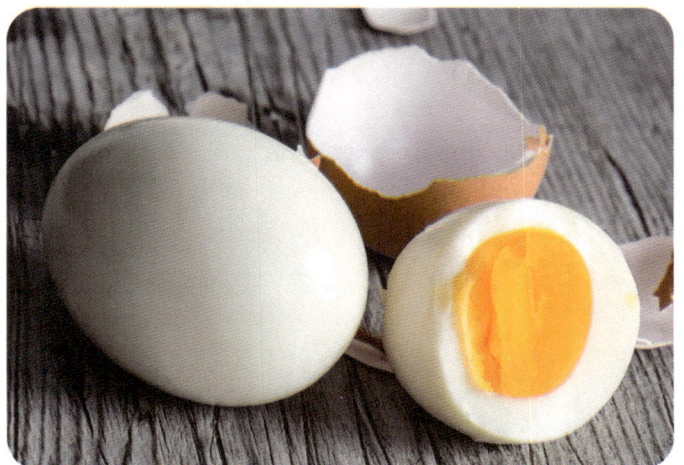

Dinner Recipes

Pork Meatloaf

Serves: 4
Cooking time: 1 & 1/2 hours
Meal: Dinner

Ingredients

1 pound frozen chopped spinach
1 tablespoon Ghee or fat of choice
½ cup finely chopped medium onion
½ pound cremini mushrooms, finely chopped
½ cup chopped celery
½ cup loosely-packed fresh Italian parsley leaves
¼ cup coconut cream
1 pound ground pork
¼ cup coconut flour
1 teaspoon kosher salt, plus more as needed
1½ teaspoons freshly-ground black pepper, plus
more as needed
¼ teaspoon freshly grated nutmeg
1 medium garlic clove, minced
2 large pastured eggs, lightly beaten
5 slices thick-cut bacon
Tomato sauce, warmed, for serving (optional)

Instructions

Heat oven to 350 degrees. Place thawed spinach
into colander and squeeze excess liquid. Sauté
onion, mushrooms, with ghee until liquid evaporated.
Toss celery and parsley into blender cup with
coconut cream, puree until smooth. In bowl, break
up pork, add spinach, coconut flour, with salt,
pepper, microplane-grated nutmeg, garlic. Add
mushroom and onion mix with slightly beaten egg
over the rest of the ingredients. Add green blended
mixture and combine ingredients into 9x5 in pan
loaf. Layer bacon on top. Bake for 70 minutes,
rotating halfway. Broil for 3 minutes. Rest loaf for
20 minutes. Top with optional tomato sauce.

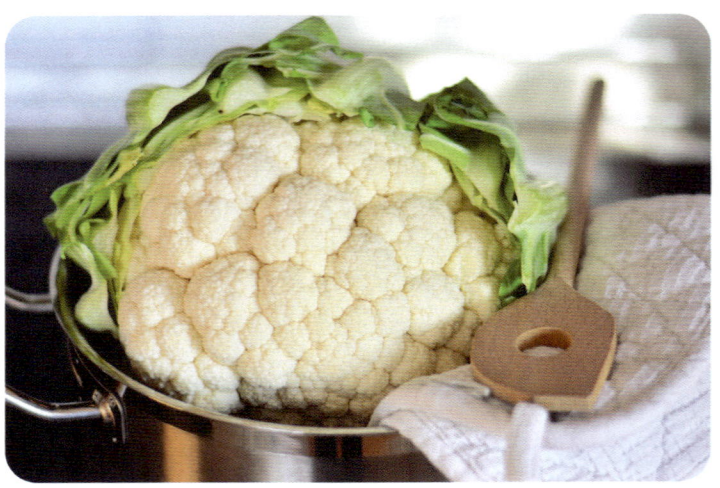

Coconut Lamb with Cauliflower Rice

Serves: 4
Cooking time: 45 minutes
Meal: Dinner

Ingredients

1 tbsp coconut oil
1 lb lamb tenderloin cubed
½ med onion
1 large carrot
4 medium tomatoes, diced
2 medium zucchini slices
1 cans of coconut milk, full fat
3 tbsp cilantro
salt and pepper
Cauliflower Rice
2 tbsp coconut oil or MCT oil
1 tbsp optional seasonings (salt, pepper, garlic,
ginger)

Instructions

To cook lamb – Cube lamb and prepare the
vegetables. Over med-high heat, melt coconut oil,
add onions and carrots. Cook until onions are
translucent. Add lamb, tomatoes, coconut milk.
Simmer for 20-30 minutes, while preparing
cauliflower rice. Add zucchini and continue to simmer
for 5-10 minutes. Cauliflower Rice: add cauliflower
into food processor and pulse until a grainy rick like
consistency. Season with salt and pepper. Heat pan
with coconut or MCI oil, add cauliflower in a pan and
add additional seasonings.

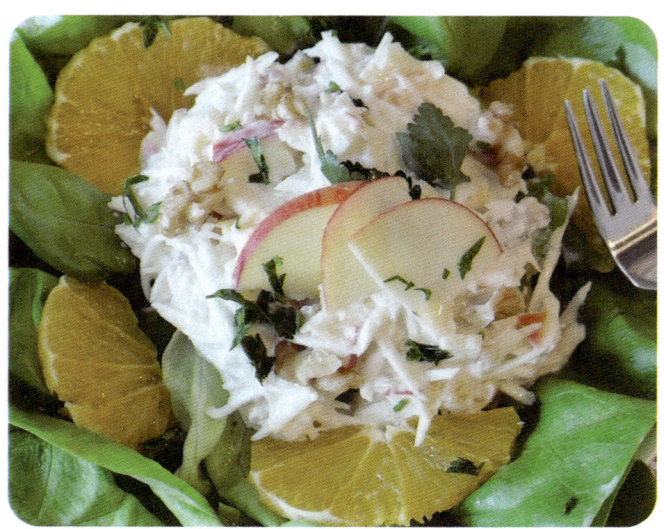

Apple Chicken Salad

Serves: 2
Cooking time: 30 minutes
Meal: Dinner

Ingredients

Salad
1 green apple diced
1 cup onion diced
1 cup grilled chicken diced
2 tsp coconut oil
1 tsp dried thyme
Salt to taste
4 cups of mixed greens

Dressing
1/2 cup extra virgin olive oil
Juice from 1 lemon
Juice from 1 orange
1/2 tsp fresh ginger, grated pinch of sea salt

Instructions

Add coconut oil to a skillet on medium heat. Add in onions and apples to skillet, cook for 10 minutes, stirring occasionally. Add in chicken, thyme, and salt. Stir all ingredients until combined Plate on a bed of mixed greens. Dressing Mix all ingredients together. Serve over salad greens or use as a marinade.

Broccoli Chicken Soup

Serves: 2
Cooking time: 40 minutes
Meal: Dinner

Ingredients

1 tbsp extra virgin olive oil
1 medium onion, chopped
Chopped chicken
2 cloves fresh garlic, crushed
2 pounds broccoli, rinsed and chopped 1 teaspoon ground thyme
salt & fresh ground pepper to taste
6-8 cups organic vegetable stock (depending on how thick) fresh chopped parsley, chives, dill

Instructions

In a large pot, heat the oil and sauté the onion and garlic until onion is soft and translucent. Add the reaming. ingredients and bring to boil. Cover, reduce heat and simmer until the broccoli is tender (about 40 minutes). Check seasoning. Puree the soup and garnish with fresh parley, chives, or dill.

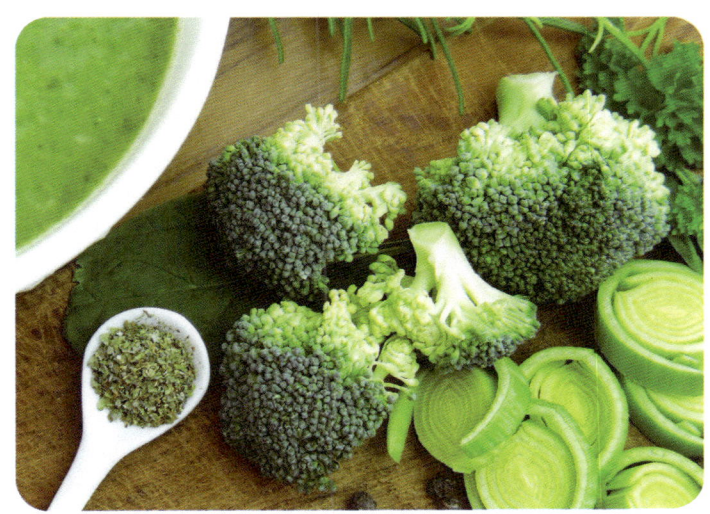

Baked Salmon With Pesto, Lemon And Dill

10 oz wild salmon filet (serves 2)

1/4 cup olive oil or MCT oil

1/2 lemon

1 tsp dill

Preheat oven to 350 degrees. Rinse salmon and pat dry with a paper towel. Rub olive oil onto the inside of a baking dish, and place salmon inside. Rub any remaining olive oil onto the salmon. Squeeze lemon onto salmon and sprinkle with dill. Bake until just done, do not over-cook. Remove from oven and top with pesto (below).

PESTO

2-3 cloves garlic, chopped

4-5 Tbsp pine nuts, almonds or walnuts

1 cup packed fresh basil leaves

1/2 cup olive oil or MCT Oil

1/2 tsp Celtic salt

Use a food processor or blender. Chop garlic. Add nuts and chop again. Add basil, chop or blend well. Feed olive oil in while machine is running. Add sea salt, taste for texture, adjust if needed.

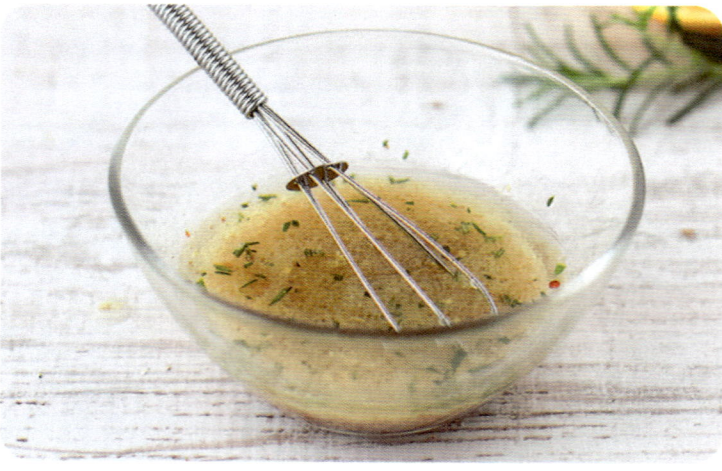

Yummy Oil And Vinegar Dressing

3 cloves garlic, crushed

1/2 cup virgin, cold pressed olive oil

1/4 cup avocado

1/4 cup apple cider vinegar

1/4 tsp Celtic or Himalayan sea salt (yes, it is important that you switch to mineralized sea salt if you currently use plain table salt)

1/4 tsp black pepper

1/2 tsp basil, oregano, and thyme

Ground Turkey Tacos

Serves: 2

Cooking time: 20 min

Meal: Dinner

Ingredients

1/2 lb ground turkey

1 medium onion

4 cloves of garlic

2 tsp coconut oil

Cilantro and onion as garnish

Avocado

Sea salt & pepper to taste

Instructions

Saute garlic and ground turkey in coconut oil. Add sea salt to taste. Assemble over lettuce leaves and add chopped green onion, cilantro, and avocado.

Chicken Stir-fry

Serves: 2

Cooking time:20 min

Meal: Dinner

Ingredients

1/4 cup veggie broth

1 pound chicken

2 cups mushrooms (try shiitake, crimini, oyster or chicken of the woods)

2 carrots, cut in matchsticks

1 teaspoon fresh grated ginger

2-3 cups chopped kale

1/4 teaspoon cayenne pepper (optional)

Wheat-free tamari or Celtic sea salt to taste

Instructions

Heat broth in a nonstick skillet over medium high heat. Add chicken, mushroom, carrots and ginger. Cook for 5 minutes. Add remaining ingredients, cook until tender. Kale should still be bright green, do not overcook.

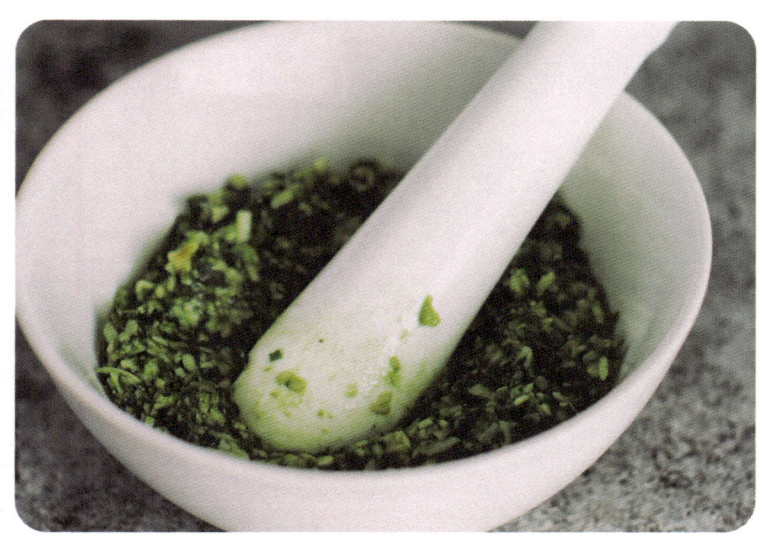

Chicken pesto

Serves: 2
Cooking time: 30 min
Meal: Dinner

Ingredients

1 4 oz. chicken breast
1-1/2 cup basil leaves
1 clove of garlic, sliced
1 tbsp. lemon juice
1/2 tsp. lemon zest
1 tbsp olive oil
2 tsp. coconut oil
salt and pepper, if desired

Instructions

Preheat oven to 425 degrees. In a food processor or blender, blend the basil and garlic, lemon juice, and grated lemon peel, slowly pour in the olive oil and mix until emulsified. Place chicken in a large rimmed baking pan, salt and pepper if desired. Coat the chicken with pesto mixture. Bake chicken until cooked thoroughly.

Sauces & Dips

Creamy herb

1/4 cup plain yogurt
1 clove garlic, peeled and minced
2 tablespoons lemon juice
2 tablespoons fresh chopped herbs (chives, parsley, basil, etc)
pinch sea salt and ground pepper

Classic vinaigrette

1/4 cup extra virgin olive oil
2 tbsp lemon juice
2 tbsp apple cider vinegar
1 teaspoon dijon mustard
pinch sea salt and ground pepper
Place all of the ingredients in a bowl and whisk to combine.

Lemon garlic *(can also be a salad dressing or marinade)*

1 cup olive oil
3 cloves garlic
4 tablespoons lemon juice
15 cracks black pepper

Creamy tarragon dressing or dip

2 tbsp. chopped tarragon
2 artichoke bottoms
1/4 cup olive oil
1 tbsp. lemon juice
Salt and pepper

Tahini dressing

1/4 cup tahini
1 1/2 Tbsp lemon juice
1 1/2 tsp apple cider vinegar
1 Tbsp freshly minced rosemary
2-3 cloves garlic minced
1 1/2 Tbsp coconut aminos
Water to thin (5-8 Tbsp
Pinch sea salt

Green Shake

1 cups of spinach
1/4 cup frozen blueberries
1 tablespoon flax oil
1 tablespoon Maca powder
1 cup almond milk

Almond Shake

6-8 oz of almond, rice, coconut or
 hemp seed milk
1 scoop protein powder
1 scoop collagen with peptides
1 scoop L-Glutamine
1 tablespoon of almond butter

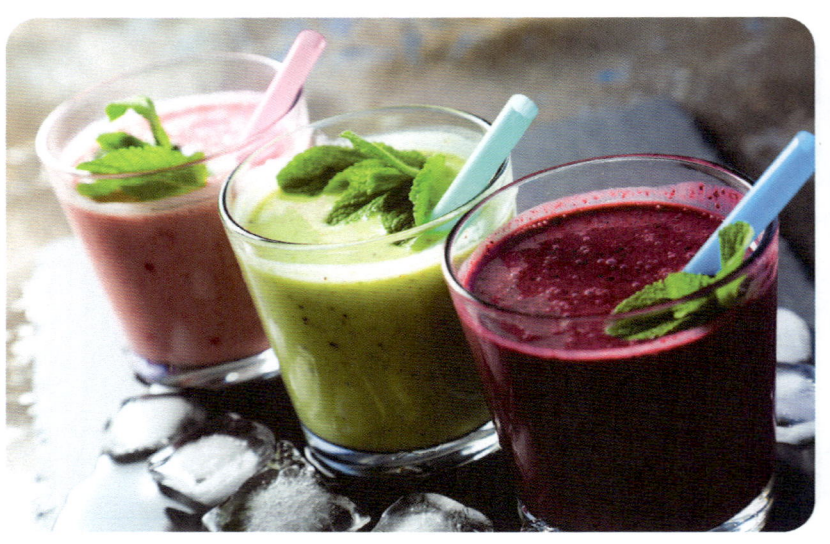

Avocado Shake

6-8 oz of almond, rice, coconut or hemp seed milk
½ avocado
1 tablespoon almond butter
1 scoop of protein powder
1 scoop of fiber (flax seeds, chia seeds, of other fiber)

Chocolate Shake

1-cup ice
1 cup almond milk
½ black tart frozen cherries
2 scoops chocolate protein powder

Blueberry Shake

6-8 oz of almond, rice, coconut or hemp seed milk
1 cup of frozen blueberries
1 teaspoon vanilla
1 scoop of protein powder
1 scoop of fiber (flax seeds, chia seeds, or other fiber)

Protein Smoothie

Protein Smoothie (serves 2):
1 cup almond or coconut milk 4 cups chopped spinach
1/2 cup frozen berries (blueberries or raspberries)
2 tablespoons nut or seed butter
1 tablespoons ground flaxseeds
4 scoops protein powder
1 teaspoon MCT Oil
ice, as needed

Protein Smoothie

Protein Smoothie (serves 2):
1 cup almond or coconut milk 4 cups chopped spinach
1/2 cup frozen berries (blueberries or raspberries)
2 tablespoons nut or seed butter
1 tablespoons ground flaxseeds
4 scoops protein powder
1 teaspoon MCT Oil
ice, as needed

Strawberry Shake

1/2 cup frozen strawberries
1 cup red chard
1 cup almond milk
2 scoops vanilla protein powder
1 cup of ice
¼ cup avocado
1 tablespoons MCT oil

Mix and Match Guide to making your own Shakes

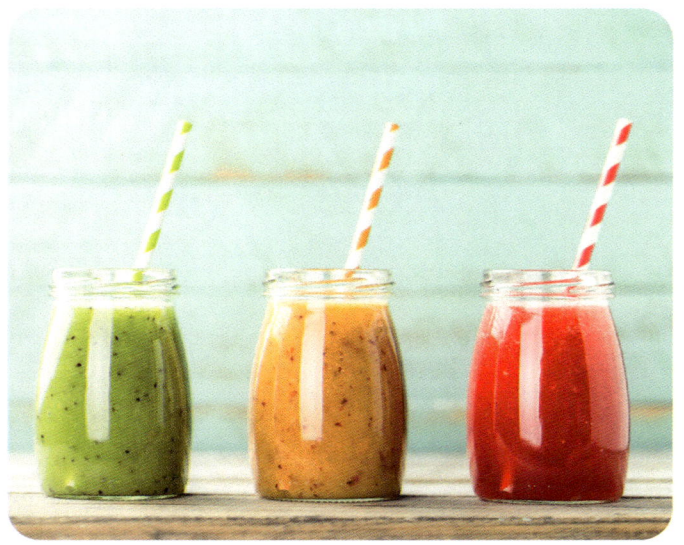

Tonic: Drink anytime/through-out the day
Apple cider vinegar/lemon/room temp water
Water with lemon or cucumber

Lemon-aid *(This will quench your sugar cravings)*
- 1 Lemon
- Water
- 1 Teaspoon of L-Glutamine powder
- 1-2 tablespoons of chia seeds (optional)
- Bone broth, homemade (or boxed at Sprouts,™ WholeFoods™ or Thrive Market™)

Cook on stove top; add spices and ginger and other herbs.

Shopping list for smoothies and shakes

Base Ingredients:
Coconut Water
Brewed herbal tea
Yerba Mate
Nut Milks
Water

Extras:
Carob
Cinnamon
Vanilla
Nutmeg
Ginger
Handfuls of greens
(kale, spinach, swiss chard)
Apples

Super foods:
Green Powder
Spirulina
Sea Salt
Maca
Acai Powder
Raw Cacao

Fats and Protein:
Nuts
Nut Milks
Rice Milk
Hemp Seed Milk
Coconut Oil
MCT Oil
Shredded Coconut
Avocado
Fax Oil
Protein Powder
(grass fed collagen, Whey, and vegetables proteins; such as pea)

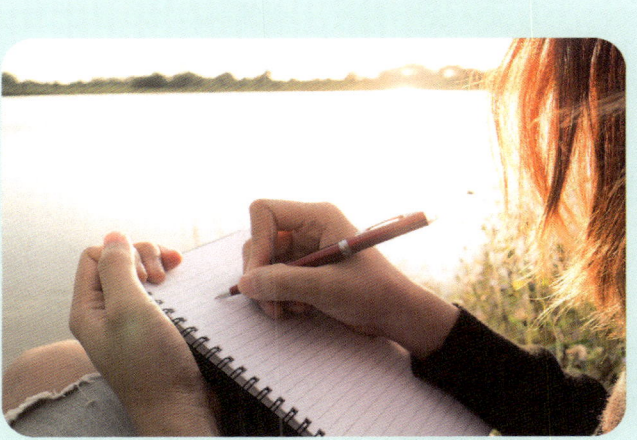

Benefit of journaling

Journaling is one way to process and articulate your thoughts and tell the "universe" what you really want.
- You worry less
- You become accountable
- It's a safe place to be honest with yourself.
- You slow down and live with intention
- Studies show on average 40% increased success with goals

The simple act of writing a few words, sentences, or paragraphs everyday can have a profound and instant effect on your life.

Daily Journal: Day 1 Date _____

WEIGHT:

Breakfast time_____   Lunch time_____

_____   _____   3 things I am thankful for today

_____   _____   _____

_____   _____   _____

_____   _____   _____

Dinner time_____   Snack time_____

_____   _____

Circle any symptoms you are noticing and to what degree, 1 being LOW, and 5 being HIGH.

Cravings	Mood
1 2 3 4 5	1 2 3 4 5

WATER

Hunger	GI Issues
1 2 3 4 5	1 2 3 4 5

OTHER DRINKS

Energy	Stress
1 2 3 4 5	1 2 3 4 5

Daily Journal: Day 2 Date _____

WEIGHT:

Breakfast time_____   Lunch time_____

_____   _____   3 things I am thankful for today

_____   _____   _____

_____   _____   _____

_____   _____   _____

Dinner time_____   Snack time_____

_____   _____

Circle any symptoms you are noticing and to what degree, 1 being LOW, and 5 being HIGH.

Cravings	Mood
1 2 3 4 5	1 2 3 4 5

WATER

Hunger	GI Issues
1 2 3 4 5	1 2 3 4 5

OTHER DRINKS

Energy	Stress
1 2 3 4 5	1 2 3 4 5

Daily Journal:

Day 3 Date _____

Breakfast time_____

_____
_____
_____
_____

Lunch time_____

_____
_____
_____
_____

WEIGHT:

3 things I am thankful for today

_____
_____
_____

Dinner time_____

_____
_____
_____
_____

Snack time_____

WATER
◯ ◯ ◯ ◯ ◯ ◯ ◯

OTHER DRINKS
◯ ◯ ◯

Circle any symptoms you are noticing and to what degree, 1 being LOW, and 5 being HIGH.

Cravings
1 2 3 4 5

Mood
1 2 3 4 5

Hunger
1 2 3 4 5

GI Issues
1 2 3 4 5

Energy
1 2 3 4 5

Stress
1 2 3 4 5

Daily Journal:

Day 4 Date _____

Breakfast time_____

_____
_____
_____
_____

Lunch time_____

_____
_____
_____
_____

WEIGHT:

3 things I am thankful for today

_____
_____
_____

Dinner time_____

_____
_____
_____

Snack time_____

WATER
◯ ◯ ◯ ◯ ◯ ◯ ◯

OTHER DRINKS
◯ ◯ ◯

Circle any symptoms you are noticing and to what degree, 1 being LOW, and 5 being HIGH.

Cravings
1 2 3 4 5

Mood
1 2 3 4 5

Hunger
1 2 3 4 5

GI Issues
1 2 3 4 5

Energy
1 2 3 4 5

Stress
1 2 3 4 5

Daily Journal:

Day 5 Date _____

WEIGHT:

Breakfast time_____

Lunch time_____

3 things I am thankful for today

_____
_____
_____
_____

Dinner time_____

Snack time_____

Circle any symptoms you are noticing and to what degree, 1 being LOW, and 5 being HIGH.

Cravings	Mood
1 2 3 4 5	1 2 3 4 5

WATER

Hunger	GI Issues
1 2 3 4 5	1 2 3 4 5

OTHER DRINKS

Energy	Stress
1 2 3 4 5	1 2 3 4 5

Daily Journal:

Day 6 Date _____

WEIGHT:

Breakfast time_____

Lunch time_____

3 things I am thankful for today

_____
_____
_____
_____

Dinner time_____

Snack time_____

Circle any symptoms you are noticing and to what degree, 1 being LOW, and 5 being HIGH.

Cravings	Mood
1 2 3 4 5	1 2 3 4 5

WATER

Hunger	GI Issues
1 2 3 4 5	1 2 3 4 5

OTHER DRINKS

Energy	Stress
1 2 3 4 5	1 2 3 4 5

Daily Journal:

Day 7   Date _____

Breakfast time_____

_____
_____
_____
_____

Lunch time_____

_____
_____
_____
_____

WEIGHT:

3 things I am thankful for today

_____
_____
_____

Dinner time_____

_____
_____
_____
_____

Snack time_____

WATER
●●●●●●●●
OTHER DRINKS
● ● ●

Circle any symptoms you are noticing and to what degree, 1 being LOW, and 5 being HIGH.

Cravings	Mood
1 2 3 4 5	1 2 3 4 5

Hunger	GI Issues
1 2 3 4 5	1 2 3 4 5

Energy	Stress
1 2 3 4 5	1 2 3 4 5

Daily Journal:

Day 8   Date _____

Breakfast time_____

_____
_____
_____
_____

Lunch time_____

_____
_____
_____
_____

WEIGHT:

3 things I am thankful for today

_____
_____
_____

Dinner time_____

_____
_____
_____
_____

Snack time_____

WATER
●●●●●●●●
OTHER DRINKS
● ● ●

Circle any symptoms you are noticing and to what degree, 1 being LOW, and 5 being HIGH.

Cravings	Mood
1 2 3 4 5	1 2 3 4 5

Hunger	GI Issues
1 2 3 4 5	1 2 3 4 5

Energy	Stress
1 2 3 4 5	1 2 3 4 5

Daily Journal:

Day 9 Date _____

WEIGHT:

Breakfast time_____

_____
_____
_____
_____

Lunch time_____

_____
_____
_____
_____

3 things I am thankful for today

_____
_____
_____

Dinner time_____

_____
_____
_____
_____

Snack time_____

WATER
● ● ● ● ● ● ● ●

OTHER DRINKS
● ● ●

Circle any symptoms you are noticing and to what degree, 1 being LOW, and 5 being HIGH.

Cravings	Mood
1 2 3 4 5	1 2 3 4 5

Hunger	GI Issues
1 2 3 4 5	1 2 3 4 5

Energy	Stress
1 2 3 4 5	1 2 3 4 5

Daily Journal:

Day 10 Date _____

WEIGHT:

Breakfast time_____

_____
_____
_____
_____

Lunch time_____

_____
_____
_____
_____

3 things I am thankful for today

_____
_____
_____

Dinner time_____

_____
_____
_____
_____

Snack time_____

WATER
● ● ● ● ● ● ● ●

OTHER DRINKS
● ● ●

Circle any symptoms you are noticing and to what degree, 1 being LOW, and 5 being HIGH.

Cravings	Mood
1 2 3 4 5	1 2 3 4 5

Hunger	GI Issues
1 2 3 4 5	1 2 3 4 5

Energy	Stress
1 2 3 4 5	1 2 3 4 5

14-DAY DETOX CLEANSE

Daily Journal:

Day 11 Date _____

WEIGHT:

Breakfast time_____
_____
_____
_____
_____

Lunch time_____
_____
_____
_____
_____

3 things I am thankful for today
_____
_____
_____

Dinner time_____
_____
_____
_____
_____

Snack time_____

WATER ● ● ● ● ● ● ● ●

OTHER DRINKS ● ● ●

Circle any symptoms you are noticing and to what degree, 1 being LOW, and 5 being HIGH.

Cravings 1 2 3 4 5   Mood 1 2 3 4 5

Hunger 1 2 3 4 5   GI Issues 1 2 3 4 5

Energy 1 2 3 4 5   Stress 1 2 3 4 5

Daily Journal:

Day 12 Date _____

WEIGHT:

Breakfast time_____
_____
_____
_____
_____

Lunch time_____
_____
_____
_____
_____

3 things I am thankful for today
_____
_____
_____

Dinner time_____
_____
_____
_____
_____

Snack time_____

WATER ● ● ● ● ● ● ● ●

OTHER DRINKS ● ● ●

Circle any symptoms you are noticing and to what degree, 1 being LOW, and 5 being HIGH.

Cravings 1 2 3 4 5   Mood 1 2 3 4 5

Hunger 1 2 3 4 5   GI Issues 1 2 3 4 5

Energy 1 2 3 4 5   Stress 1 2 3 4 5

Daily Journal:

Day 13 Date _____

Breakfast time_____

_____

_____

_____

_____

Lunch time_____

_____

_____

_____

WEIGHT:

3 things I am thankful for today

_____

_____

_____

Dinner time_____

_____

_____

_____

_____

Snack time_____

WATER
○ ○ ○ ○ ○ ○ ○ ○

OTHER DRINKS
○ ○ ○

Circle any symptoms you are noticing and to what degree, 1 being LOW, and 5 being HIGH.

Cravings
1 2 3 4 5

Mood
1 2 3 4 5

Hunger
1 2 3 4 5

GI Issues
1 2 3 4 5

Energy
1 2 3 4 5

Stress
1 2 3 4 5

Daily Journal:

Day 14 Date _____

Breakfast time_____

_____

_____

_____

_____

Lunch time_____

_____

_____

_____

WEIGHT:

3 things I am thankful for today

_____

_____

_____

Dinner time_____

_____

_____

_____

_____

Snack time_____

WATER
○ ○ ○ ○ ○ ○ ○ ○

OTHER DRINKS
○ ○ ○

Circle any symptoms you are noticing and to what degree, 1 being LOW, and 5 being HIGH.

Cravings
1 2 3 4 5

Mood
1 2 3 4 5

Hunger
1 2 3 4 5

GI Issues
1 2 3 4 5

Energy
1 2 3 4 5

Stress
1 2 3 4 5

GRASS-FED BEEF VS. GRAIN-FED / GRASS-FINISHED BEEF

WHAT'S THE DIFFERENCE?

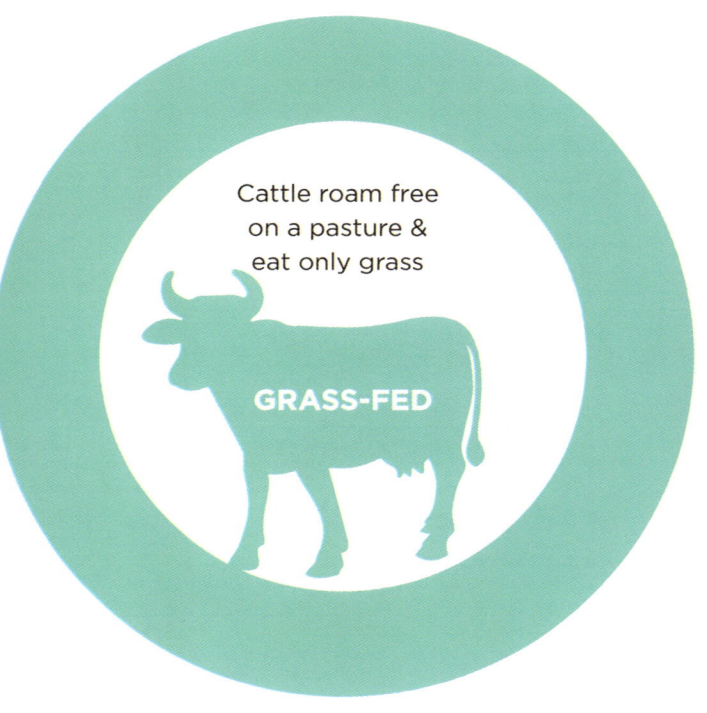

Cattle roam free on a pasture & eat only grass

GRASS-FED

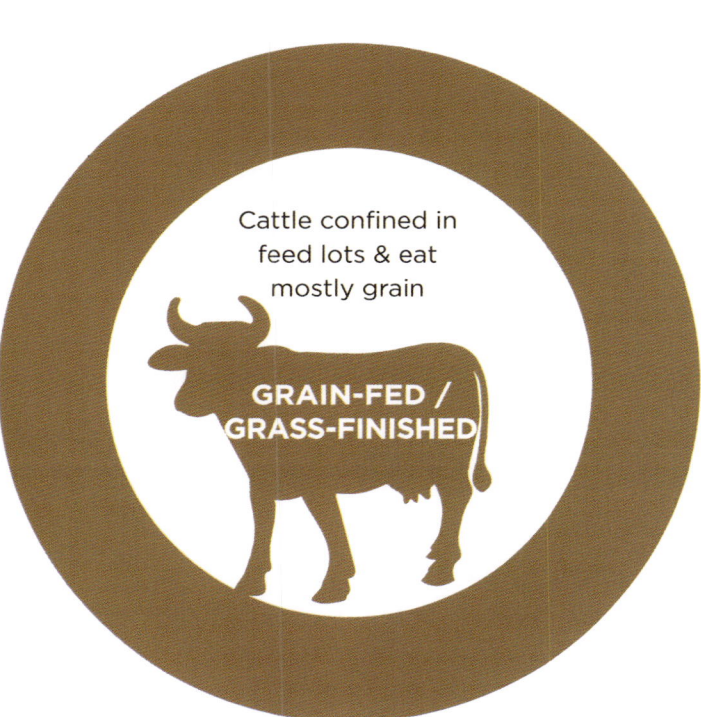

Cattle confined in feed lots & eat mostly grain

GRAIN-FED / GRASS-FINISHED

- Meat that is hormone and antibiotic free
- Leaner and juicier, thanks to higher moisture content
- Rich in omega-3 fatty acids, vitamin B6 & beta carotene
- As little as 140 calories per serving
- Lower cholesterol

- Added hormone and antibiotics
- Greasy, not juicy
- "Fattened up" on a variety of grain or corn by-products which can fatten us up
- Regular consumption not recommended as part of a healthy diet
- Higher cholesterol

Foods To Avoid During A Sugar Detox

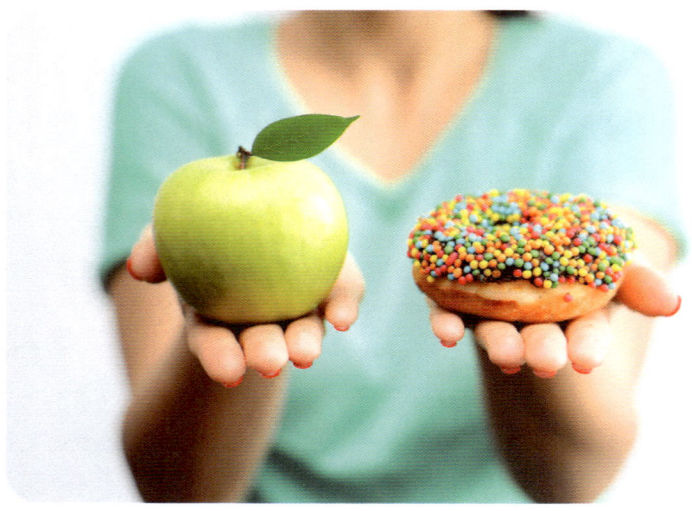

Vegetables
- Corn
- Soybeans

Fruit
- Excessive; fresh and dried

Dairy
- Cheese
- Milk
- Cream or creamer
- Half & half
- Sour cream

Condiments
- Ketchup
- BBQ sauce
- Balsamic vinegar
- Store bought mayonnaise
- Soy sauce (contains wheat)
- Tomato sauce with added sugar

Sweeteners
- Natural and artificial
- Products that list sugar free

Beverages
- Alcohol
- Fruit juice
- Soda
- Coffee shakes or drinks
- Fruit smoothies
- Energy drinks
- Protein shakes with added sugars

Refined Foods
- Bread
- Cake
- Cookies
- Brownies
- Cereal
- Chips
- Crackers
- Pretzels
- Muffins
- Cupcakes
- White flour pasta
- White flour pizza
- White flour and corn tortillas

Grains/Legumes
- Arrowroot
- Barley
- Couscous
- White flour
- Rice
- Rye
- Spelt
- Wheat
- Processed flours
- Excess beans & legumes
- Popcorn

How to read a label

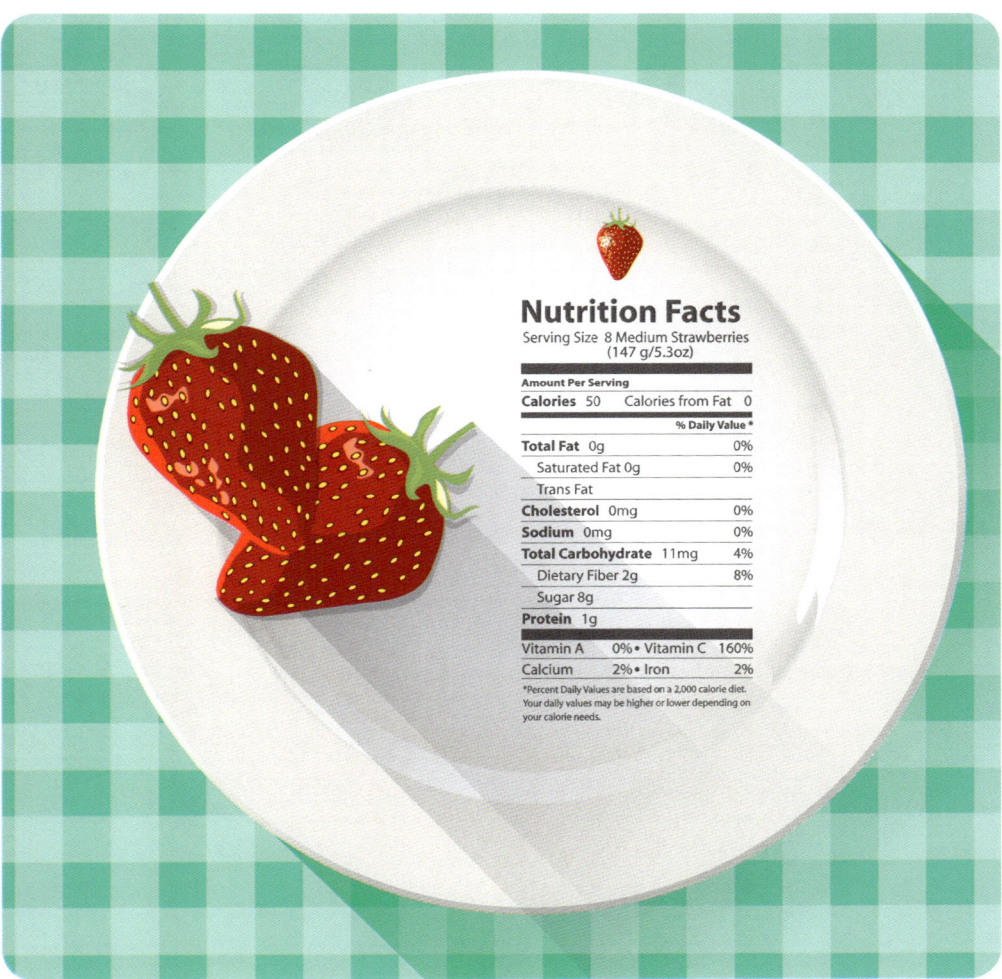

Nutrition Facts

Serving Size 8 Medium Strawberries
(147 g/5.3oz)

Amount Per Serving

Calories 50	Calories from Fat	0

	% Daily Value *
Total Fat 0g	0%
Saturated Fat 0g	0%
Trans Fat	
Cholesterol 0mg	0%
Sodium 0mg	0%
Total Carbohydrate 11mg	4%
Dietary Fiber 2g	8%
Sugar 8g	
Protein 1g	

Vitamin A	0%	Vitamin C	160%
Calcium	2%	Iron	2%

*Percent Daily Values are based on a 2,000 calorie diet.
Your daily values may be higher or lower depending on
your calorie needs.

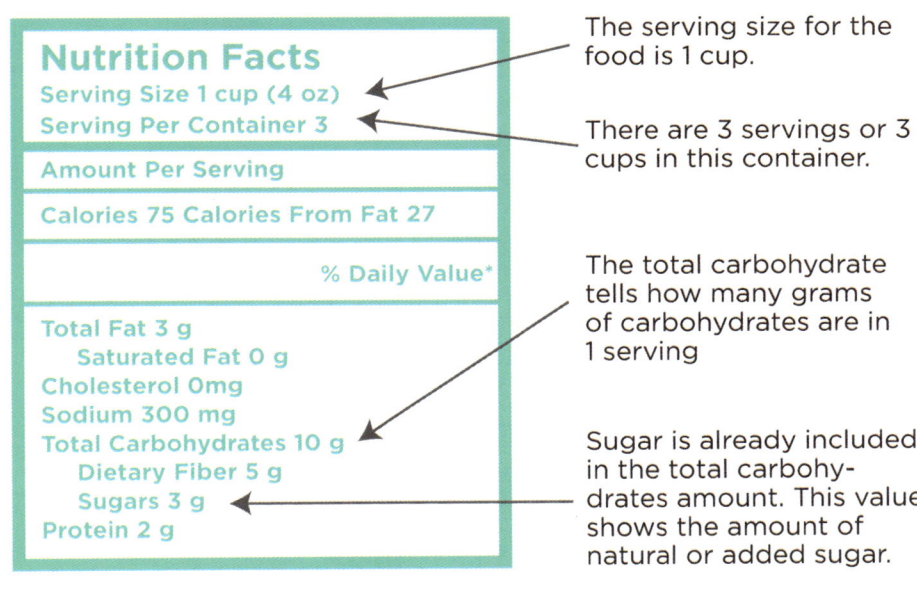

Nutrition Facts

Serving Size 1 cup (4 oz)
Serving Per Container 3

Amount Per Serving

Calories 75 Calories From Fat 27

% Daily Value*

Total Fat 3 g
   Saturated Fat 0 g
Cholesterol 0mg
Sodium 300 mg
Total Carbohydrates 10 g
   Dietary Fiber 5 g
   Sugars 3 g
Protein 2 g

The serving size for the food is 1 cup.

There are 3 servings or 3 cups in this container.

The total carbohydrate tells how many grams of carbohydrates are in 1 serving

Sugar is already included in the total carbohydrates amount. This value shows the amount of natural or added sugar.

Sugar is NOT healthy

Sugar intake is at the highest all time levels. Sugar is the key player in making your fat and sick. Excess sugar consumption has been associated with obesity, type 2 diabetes, cardiovascular disease, certain types of cancer, tooth decay, non-alcoholic fatty liver, accelerated aging, depression, cognitive decline and a lot more health issues.

Focus on eating no more than 25 grams of added sugar per day, for women and children, 35 grams for men. Focusing on preparing healthy meals and be aware of what you put into your body. Chose wisely, remember your WHY, your goals.

The more you monitor your sugar intake the less likely you will have sugar cravings, the easier it will be to lose weight and have energy.

The majority of blood sugar issues are reversible and preventable. Did you know that sugar is 8 times as addictive as cocaine?

What's interesting is while cocaine and heroin activate only one spot for pleasure in the brain, sugar lights up the brain like a pinball machine.
Dr. Mark Hyman

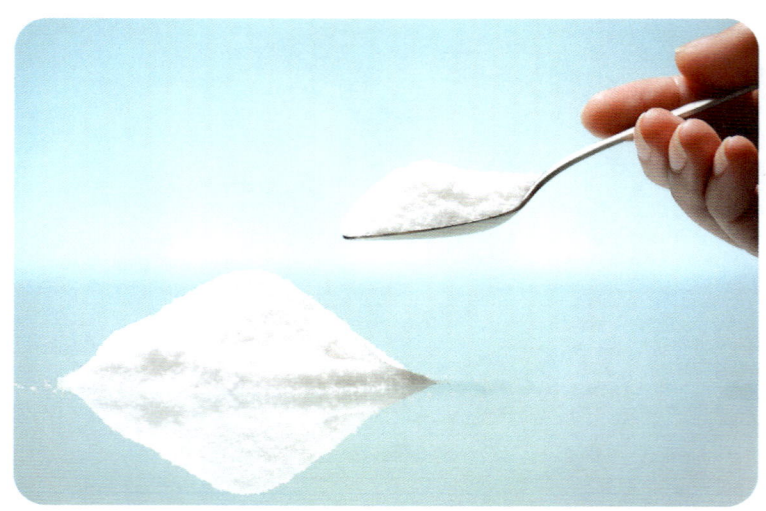

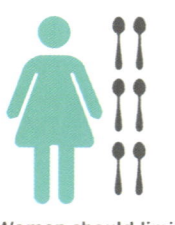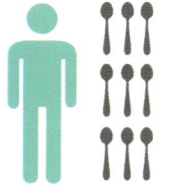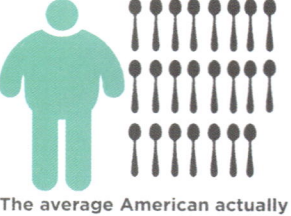

Women should limit added sugar to 100 calories per day or about 6 teaspoons.

Men should limit added sugar to 150 calories per day or about 9 teaspoons.

The average American actually consumes 365 calories per day or about 23 teaspoons.

How much sugar is too much?

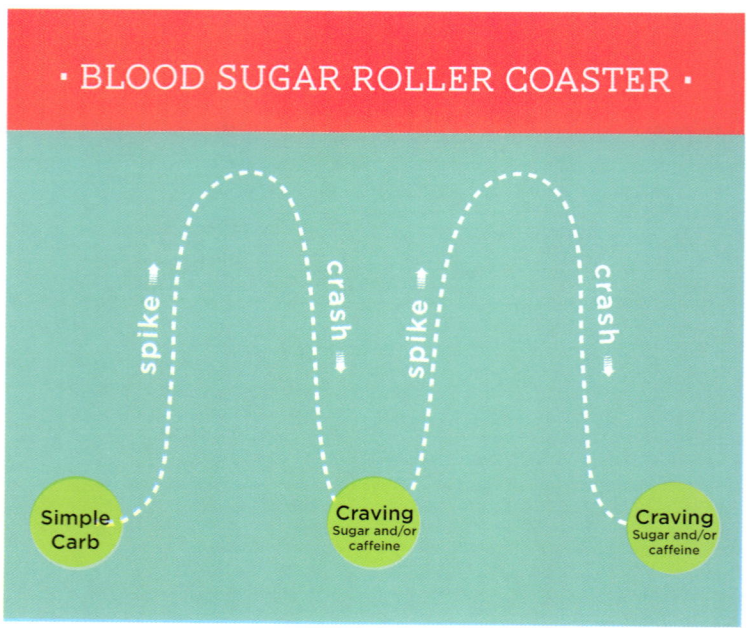

· BLOOD SUGAR ROLLER COASTER ·

spike · crash · spike · crash

Simple Carb

Craving Sugar and/or caffeine

Craving Sugar and/or caffeine

Hidden Sugars

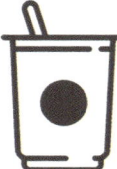

Yoplait® Strawberry Yogurt contains 18 grams of sugar.

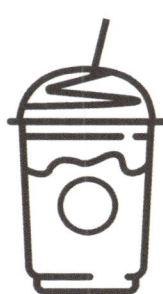

One Starbucks® Mocha Grande Frappuccino contains 61 grams of sugar.

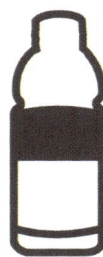

Vitamin Water® contains 32 grams of sugar in a 20 ounce bottle.

Kellogg's® Raisin Bran Omega 3 from Flaxseed Cereal
(sounds healthy right?)
contains 17 grams of sugar .

After every meal ask yourself:

- Do I have blood sugar crashes during the day? Yes / No
- Do I crave sweets or carbohydrates during the afternoon or evening? Yes / No
- Do I get a full night's rest? Yes / No
- Do I have enough mental energy to get me through the day? Yes / No
- Am I tired after eating a meal? Yes / No
- Do I crave sugar right after a meal? Yes / No
- Can I go 4-6 hours between meals? Yes / No

If you have any of the above symptoms then your blood sugar is not balanced. Sugar affects our moods and can cause anxiety, depression and irritability and makes it harder for us to manage stress. The goal is to balance your blood sugar by staying in the green zone.

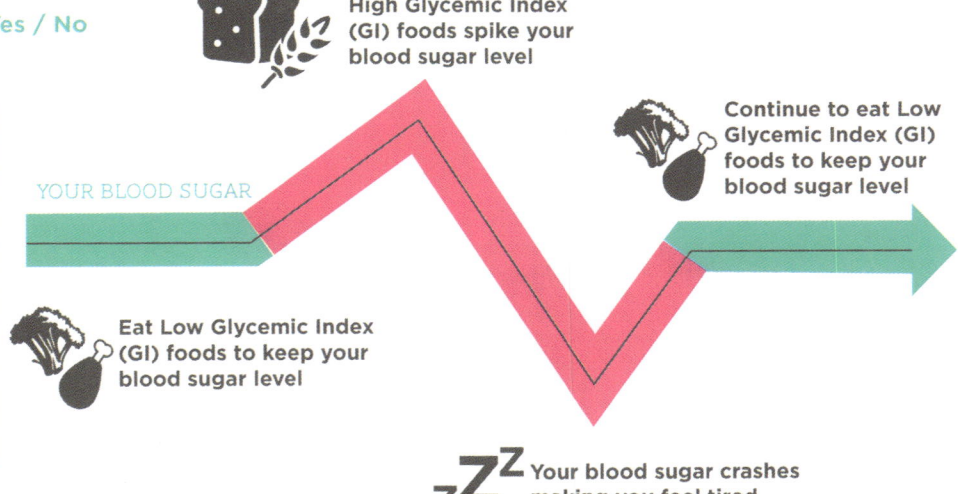

High Glycemic Index (GI) foods spike your blood sugar level

Continue to eat Low Glycemic Index (GI) foods to keep your blood sugar level

YOUR BLOOD SUGAR

Eat Low Glycemic Index (GI) foods to keep your blood sugar level

zZᶻ Your blood sugar crashes making you feel tired

Dry-skin brushing benefits:

■ By stimulating your lymphatic system and helping it release toxins, dry skin brushing is a powerful detoxification aid.
Your lymphatic system is responsible for eliminating cellular waste products. Lymphatic congestion is a major factor leading to inflammation and disease.

■ Dry skin brushing removes dead dry skin, improving appearance, clearing your clogged pores, and allowing your skin to "breathe."

■ When you dry brush your skin, it increases circulation to your skin, which encourages the elimination of metabolic waste.

■ Dry skin brushing may help to diminish the appearance of cellulite.

■ The act of dry brushing has been described as meditative, **stress relieving** and has been compared to a light wholebody massage.

■ Dry skin brushing may help support your digestion, organs and kidney function.

■ It's invigorating! Along with glowing and tighter skin, regular dry skin brushers report feeling invigorated. Use gentle pressure while brushing (toward your heart).

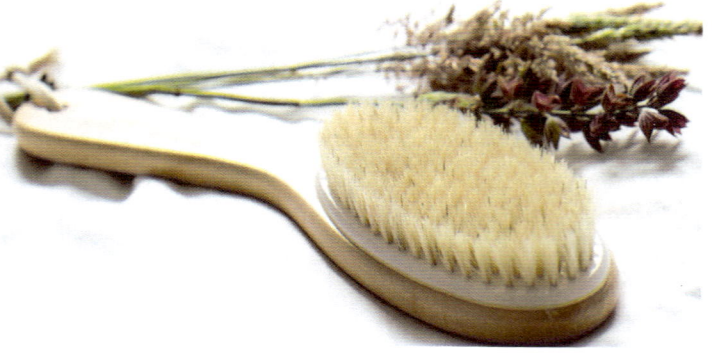

Stress

Stress is a normal adaptive coping response that has evolved over hundreds of millions of years. Chronic stress occurs when modern life exposes us to stress constantly –multitasking, juggling or moving too quickly - our bodies are not designed to be stressed 10 hours a day with no breaks.

Chronic stress symptoms can affect your body, your thoughts and your feelings and your behavior. Stress unchecked will contribute to health problems like:

■ High-blood pressure

■ Heart disease

■ Obesity

■ Diabetes

■ Depression

■ Aging prematurely

Tools to live by:

■ Turn down the intensity – emotional reaction

■ Rest

■ Good nutrition

■ Meditation

■ Exercise

■ Being positive

■ Connect

■ Exhale longer – Breathe deeper

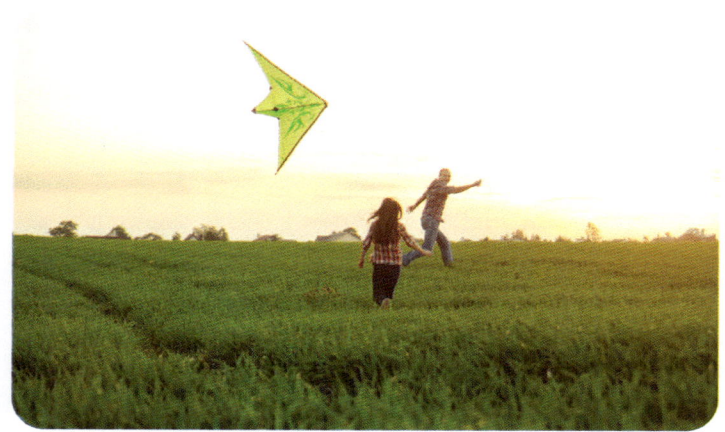

Mouvement and exercise

Our bodies are built to move and if you find yourself sitting all day, or even part of your day, you need to get up and move. Put a timer on for at least every hour and get up and walk around the block or take an exercise class during you lunch hour. Try walking at least 30 minutes each night after dinner. Studies have proven that being sedentary during the day puts you at risk of:

- Having a low metabolism
- Increasing the chances of back pain
- A drop in the levels of healthy cholesterol
- Cardiovascular diseases associated with obesity
- Organ damage, brain damage
- Developing posture problems
- Muscle degeneration
- Leg disorders such as viscous veins and weak bones

Benefit of daily movement
- Healthy body weight
- Improved metabolism (digestion)
- Disease prevention
- Strong body immunity
- Increase in bone density
- Cardiovascular health
- Stress reduction
- Pain management
- Body rehabilitation

Remove sitting in chairs - Simple but tough to actually put into practice for most. Prove me wrong! Sit less in chairs and learn to squat and sit on the floor instead. We should be able to sit on the floor in various positions without feeling pain.

Find out what movement means to you - Enjoy movement for its own sake instead of external rewards.

Make movement a priority - turn your movement into your passion.

Movement - Move more. Fit in movement into your life, into your job your life. Prevention is better than cure. Push yourself to do something that gets you out of your comfort zone. Do not think about it too much.

What are you training for?
Gain Muscles? Get lean? Lose weight? maybe an event?

Embodiment - Use movement to reconnect with your body and mind and bring the body back into experiencing things.

Love being in nature. Move in nature. We are designed to be exposed to and move in all sorts of natural environments. Touch the world with your senses - go barefoot, dig in dirt and even hug a tree.

Be strong, to be useful - So once you've improved yourself, that's great and all but now what? Personal self striving alone can become stagnant and meaningless if you do not help those around you. After you have focused within, turn your attention outward to help others.You family/tribe, your community, the environment - the world. Once you have "changed your body" what will you do to "change the world"?

Play - with your children, with an adult, by yourself. Play has many forms. Most are afraid or conditioned to not see it's importance. Are you play deprived? When's the last time you wrestled, played tag or hide and seek. It is far from a waste of time. "Play like your life depended on it".

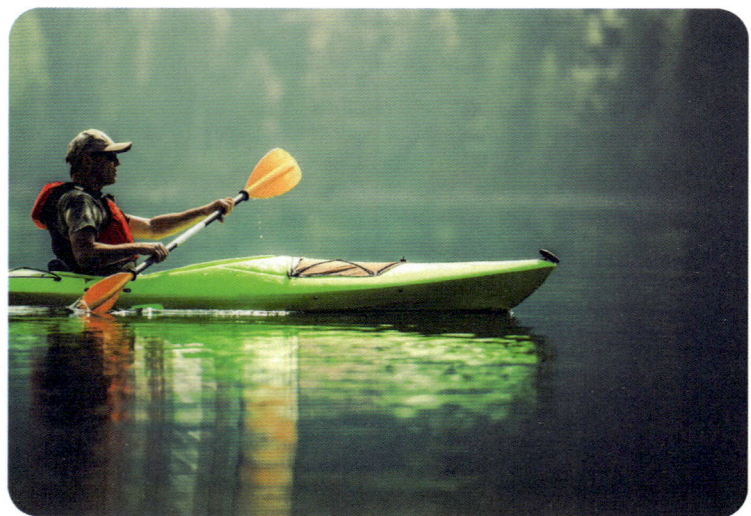

What can you do?

Ideas for outdoor experiences:

1. Walking
2. Running
3. Rollerblading/rollerskating
4. Bike riding
5. Hiking
6. Skateboarding
7. Swimming
8. Kayaking
9. Sports - tennis, soccer, basketball, beach volleyball, etc.
10. Canoeing
11. Gardening
12. Trail running
13. Walking the dog
14. Horseback riding
15. Aerobics
16. Frisbee
17. Sailing
18. Home repairs
19. Uphill sprinting
20. Windsurfing
21. Lawn mowing
22. Sight seeing walking trails/tours
23. Tai chi
24. Scuba diving
25. Washing a car
26. Snorkeling
27. Fishing
28. Surfing
29. Trampoline
30. Fly a kite
31. Water aerobics
32. Rowing
33. Water polo
34. Water skiing
35. Rock climbing
36. Mountain biking
37. Outdoor yoga
38. Rollerskiing [1]
39. Stand-up paddelboard
40. Trapeze

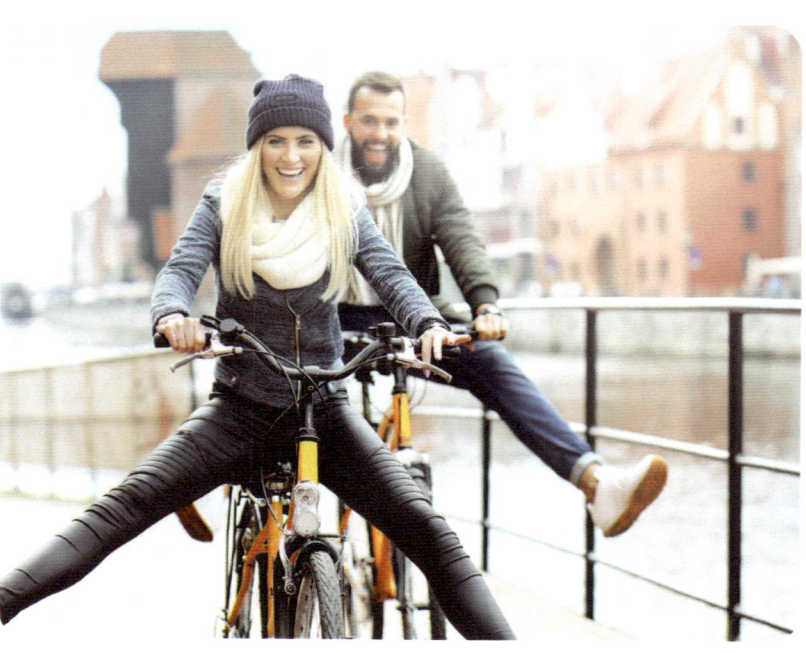

Sleep

Sleep not only makes us feel better but it is important for our overall health. Adequate sleep is a key player for a healthy heart, weight and mind.

Getting enough sleep improves your memory and will help you perform better after a good night's sleep. Not enough sleep will shorten your lifespan. Recent studies show that women who get less than five hours of sleep consistently have a shorter life span. Inflammation is linked to heart disease, stroke, diabetes and arthritis and premature aging, research indicates that people with less sleep have higher blood levels of inflammatory proteins than those who get more sleep.

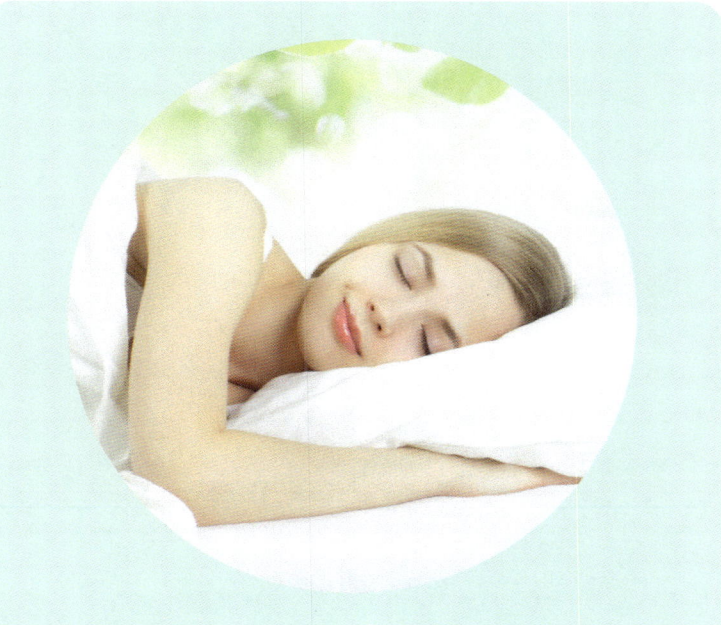

Sleep, Sleep...

Sleep is a vital indicator of overall health and well being. We spend 1/3 of our lives sleeping. It is so important to get enough sleep every night. Not getting enough sleep not only makes our minds less alert, but our bodies too and also slows down our metabolism. Our bodies need somewhere between 7- 8 hours of sleep every night.

Take this quick sleep quiz:

Do you sleep less than 9 hour per night? **Yes / No**

Do you have problems falling asleep or staying asleep? **Yes / No**

Do you wake up more exhausted than when you went to bed? **Yes / No**

Do you have fat around your midsection, despite your watching your food intake? **Yes / No**

Have you experienced memory problems? **Yes / No**

If you answered YES to the majority of these questions, you probably need more sleep.

Reintroduce foods back into your diet

After the 14 days, reintroduce foods you have eliminated. The purpose of this process is to identify what your body can handle and what it can't handle.These are foods that cause inflammation, irritation and digestive issues. Most of the time you will have some sort of triggers even before starting this program without realizing it.

During this process you will reintroduce gluten and dairy, but one at a time. It is important to isolate one food to determine if it is one of the foods that creates a reaction the next day.

You will continue on the program (detox cleanse) and eating all the good foods from the last 14 days, but you will be adding gluten to see if you react. Reintroduce gluten 2 to 3 times a day for 2 days and journal any reactions.

Daily Questions:

- Does anything happen immediately after eating gluten: such as running nose or mucus, feeling tired or headaches?
- How is your energy level?
- Did you have a healthy bowel movement?
- Did you sleep poorly?
- Did you feel angry, moody or irritable?
- Did you have brain fog?
- Did you gain weight immediately?

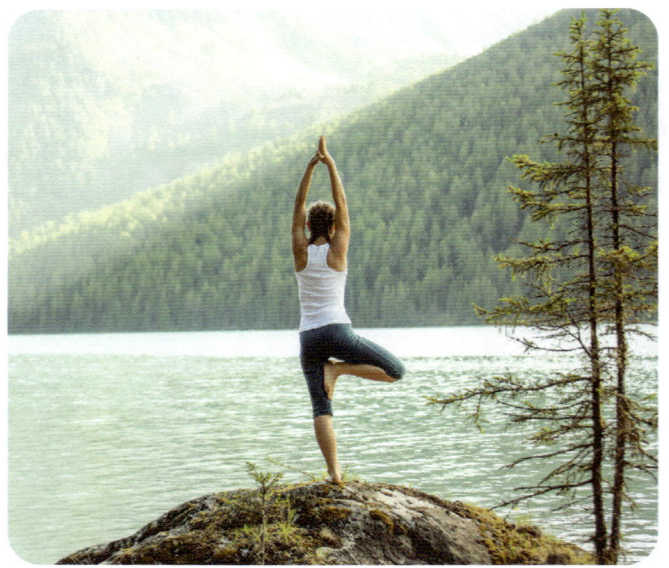

If you have any of these adverse reactions then you might need to eliminate those foods from your diet completely. If you reactions are mild, then you might want to only eat these foods more infrequently.

There is no need to be black and white with the way you are eating for the rest of your life. If you are going to eat something you know is not good for you, enjoy it. Be kind to yourself and try to notice if you feel guilty.

It is very important to notice a strong connection between what you eat and what you feel. This is a process, and connecting internally with how you feel and creating a lifestyle you love is a formula for a happier life. That is a place where we can be more creative, come up with ideas, find our passions and love life to the fullest.

Q & As

Organic: Why? Non-organic produce contains pesticides and herbicides that overwork your liver and increase toxicity in the body. Organic foods are more nutritious than non-organic foods which means you'll be satisfied with less food so you'll feel light, yet energized after eating. Although organic foods tend to cost more, you're worth it, especially during your cleanse!

Will I lose weight? Yes, most likely you will lose some excess weight when you avoid processed sugar, gluten, dairy and other food irritants.

Cravings: Consume alkalizing foods such as dark green leafy vegetables. In a few days these cravings will pass.

Emotional imbalance: Sometimes cravings for sweet flavor is an indication we're yearning for more sweetness in our lives. Consider what you might really be needing?

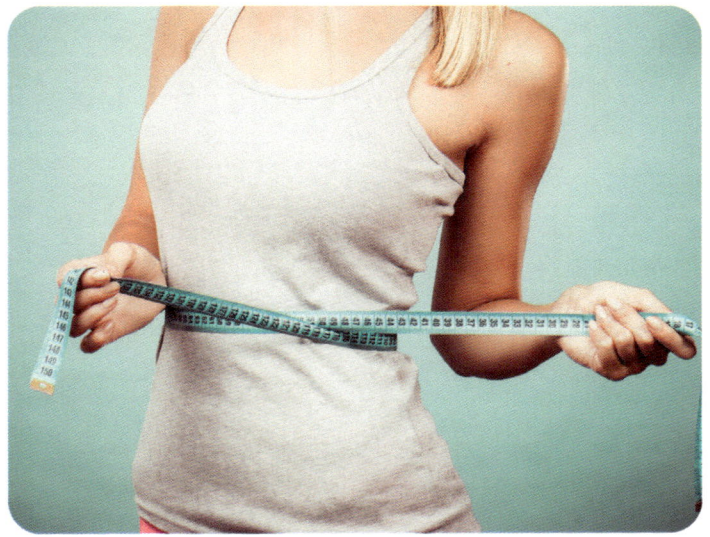

Can I take my regular supplements and medications?

It is always best to consult with your healthcare provider before starting any detox cleanse.

What if I get constipated:

■ Use a laxative tea.

■ Home Enema: Enemas can be a life-saver during a cleanse. Hold the water in for as long as you can before eliminating.

■ Colonic: This treatment is done by trained technicians at a colon hydrotherapy center.

■ Magnesium Citrate promotes healthy bowel function. Take 2-3 capsules 2x/day until your bowels start moving again. If you have loose stool or diarrhea, reduce the amount.

What are the benefits of detox cleanse?

The effects of detox cleanse vary from person to person. There is no one way to determine how a cleanse will affect you before you do it. Once you get over the uncomfortable withdrawals from sugar, caffeine or alcohol, you will start to feel better with more energy, improved digestion, clearer skin and an enhanced sense of well-being. Also, this program is a great way to jump start your way to an all around healthier lifestyle. Slowly you will integrate the tips, meal plans and recipes into your normal routine.

How do I know if I need to detox / cleanse?

You probably need a detox cleans when you feel you body is not functioning at it's best, when you feel tired, you have gained weight, you do not have enough energy to get through the day or you have mood swings. Our bodies detox naturally, but after constant exposure to toxins, chronic stress, poor eating, poor sleep and no movement it is hard for our bodies to heal.

Do I have to give up coffee and wine?

Unfortuately yes, both coffee and wine make it difficult for your liver to heal. You might want to wean yourself off coffee and wine a couple weeks prior to starting this program.

Testimonials

"My weight this morning was 185.8! I'm seriously more than shocked! I remember the first day of the program, I was so embarrassed when it came to weighing and measuring myself! But now it feels great to see the huge difference —49 lbs loss since mid-January! But more importantly, I got my before and after blood work results from Courtney yesterday and it actually gave me tears of joy for all of my efforts! I really had big doubts to ever even be this close to a goal that I put out to the universe of 175 lbs! I hope you realize your role in this process! Your faith, encouragement, support and love for your work made a HUGE difference, oh Courtney too! I will continue to thank you, Melissa, for probably the rest of my life, for being such an inspiration and influence in my life! Thank you!!!"

L. Romo ~ San Diego

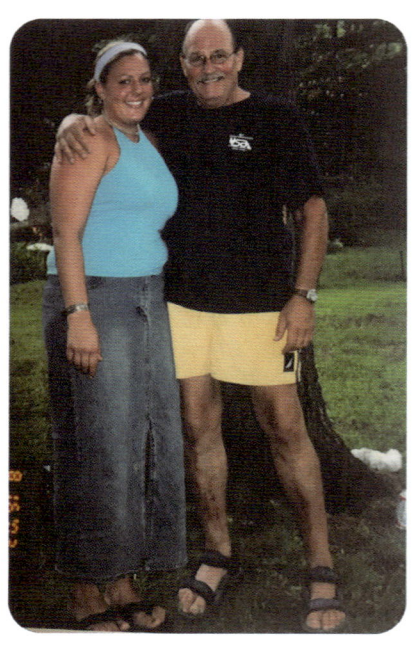

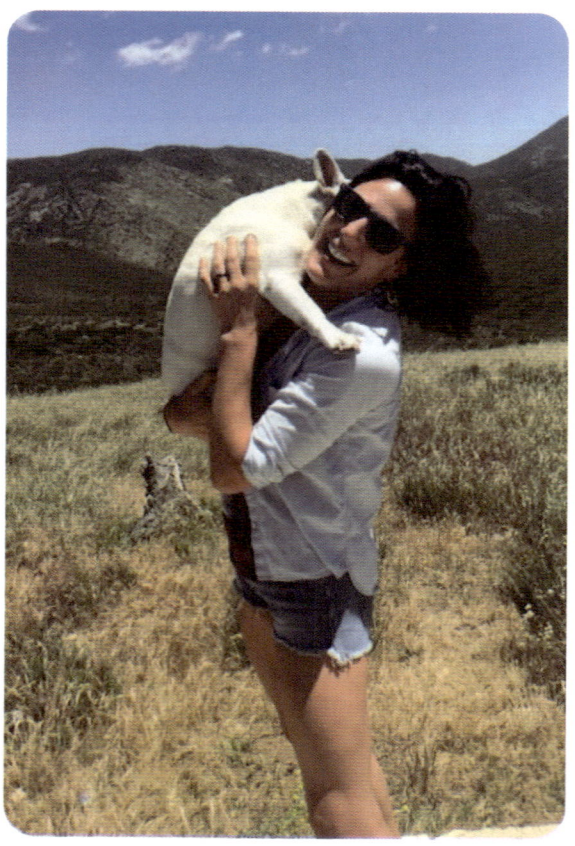

"I have been working with Melissa, for now, two years! It has been not only a beautiful process getting to know her as a person/-coach, BUT it has also been the most transformational for my physical body and self-growth within the past two years. She has a magic way of "digging deep" emotionally with me and allowing me to be my most authentic self. I consider myself to be a quite intuitive person and reading people, but Melissa is incredibly intuitive when it comes to how I am feeling and what is bothering me. She gives me that space to unload, so I can release and move forward, instead of getting "stuck" and/or stagnant in both my relationships or career path. She has become a very important person in my life and I have learned SO much from her! I have lost weight both on the scale but a lot of emotional weight which has been a life changer for me. I did her 6- week sugar cleanse and received coaching from her throughout and that is what really helped. I had amazing results all around. More clarity in my mind, less anxiety, clearer skin and way less inflammation in my whole body. I continued on after her 6-weeks cleanses and created a lifestyle for myself opposed to a diet. Melissa is a beautiful soul both inside and out and she will be a lifelong friend as well as someone who helped me become my best self. Thank you, Melissa!"

K. Lucek, San Diego, CA

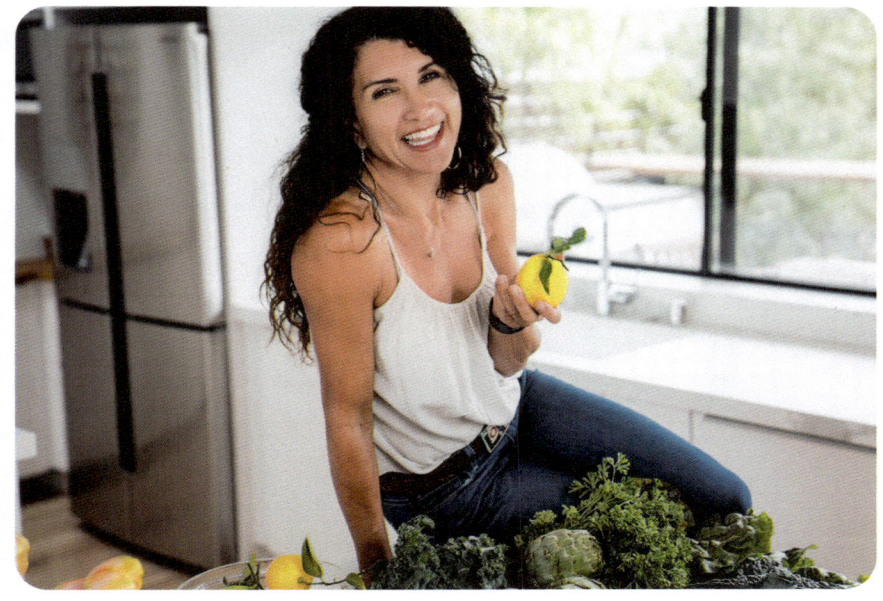

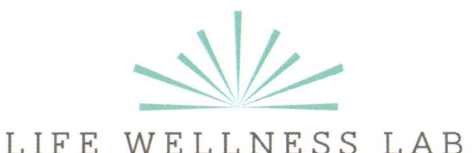

LIFE WELLNESS LAB

CREDIBILITY

My name is Melissa McLane, founder of **Life Wellness Lab**. If you are inspired by feeling more energetic, looking and feeling your best, and pointing your life in a happy and healthful direction, all with the help of a gentle and encouraging guide, then you're in the right place. I'm here to help, and so glad you're here!

MISSION

My whole-life programs at **Life Wellness Lab** have one mission: To completely transform your health, well-being and happiness through my integrated vision of diet, nutrition and lifestyle.

THOUGHT LEADER/PHILOSOPHY/CORE BELIEF

My program has transformed the lives of many and my philosophy has always been to assist the total person. This means helping you change your body chemistry, living a more active lifestyle and helping you to get "un-stuck" and living your full potential.

EPIPHANY

When I was pregnant with my first child, I was diagnosed with thyroid cancer. I needed surgery immediately and though I was blessed with a healthy daughter, I knew I had to look at what was causing me to be unhealthy. Marketers and big business inundate us with diets, exercise programs, supplements; all with the promise of a better, healthier you. I know, by my personal experience and that of my clients, it takes more than a pill or a gym. It's the collective life that makes you!

PROMISE

If there's anything I want to leave you with, it's that there's hope. You may have struggled for years with low energy, extra weight, sugar addiction. The mental barriers to break through these issues are no doubt, tough for you.

REASONS TO BELIEVE

For the last 15 years, I've coached hundreds of people through tough emotional, occupational and mindset difficulties. I found that first addressing health issues had a trickling effect that made other life issues easier to manage. The change in mindset and better health and lifestyle has a tremendous effect on total health.

COMMITMENT

My life's work is to assist and guide as many people as I can to healthy, happy and fulfilled lives. I know how to do this for you so welcome, and let's get started today!

Here is to YOUR beautiful life!

Melissa

99790511R00031

Made in the USA
Columbia, SC
11 July 2018